COOS COOPERATIVE

3 2881 00683158 5

S0-ACK-457

2001

DATE DUE

JUL - 6 2002	
OCT 1 5 2002	
MAR 2 9 2006	
JUL 7 2008	
NOV 3 0 2009	
12-21-09	
01-07-10	
FEB 1 3 2017	

L

Lo

Nat

!

DEMCO, INC. 38-2931

COQUILLE PUBLIC LIBRARY
105 N. BIRCH
COQUILLE, OR 97423

Disclaimer:
Before beginning any exercise program consult your physician. The author and the publisher disclaim any liability, personal or professional, resulting from the application or misapplication of any of the information in this publication.

Live Long, Look Young!
Text copyright © 2001 by Lisa Trivell
Photos copyright © 2001 The Hatherleigh Company, Ltd.

All rights reserved. No part of this book may be reproduced in any form or by any means, electronic or mechanical, including photocopying, recording, or by any information storage and retrieval system, without permission in writing from the publisher.

Hatherleigh Press
An Affiliate of W.W. Norton & Company, Inc.
5-22 46th Avenue, Suite 200
Long Island City, NY 11101
1-800-528-2550

This edition is printed on acid-free paper that meets the American National Standards Institute z39-48 Standard.

Library of Congress Cataloging-in-Publication Data available upon request.
ISBN 1-57826-059-0

Cover design by Angel Harleycat
Interior Design by Fatema Tarzi
Photographs by Peter Field Peck

All Hatherleigh Press titles are available for bulk purchase, special promotions, and premiums. For more information, please contact the manager of our Special Sales Department at 1-800-528-2550.

Printed in Canada   10 9 8 7 6 5 4 3 2 1

Live Long, Look Young!

Natural Health and Beauty...
the Hamptons Way!

Lisa Trivell

photography by Peter Field Peck

Hatherleigh Press • New York

Acknowledgements

I would like to give special thanks to my publisher Andrew Flach who supported the idea of the I Can't Believe It's Yoga series and was key in the launching of this book.

To RoseMarie Alfieri, Fatema Tarzi and Caroline Christman for her support and editorial talent.

To Peter Field Peck, an extremely talented photographer. He understands the concept of the book and was able to capture it on film.

Thanks to all the people who participated in the book as profiles:
Frances Alenikoff, Mike Bahel, Bernard Brule, Lucia Hwong, Hedy Klineman, Kent Klineman, Vicky Magliario, Susyn Reeve, Jerry Starr, Jane Umanoff

A special thanks to all my students and friends who participated in the book as models:
Mike Bahel, Victoria Magliaro, Herb August, Mary Bailey, John Wiltshire, Sue Petykowski, Marge Goldsmith, Anne Hollister, Evelyn Konrad, Lynne Lezcia, Richard Settducati, Lucia Hwong, Annalie Dooling, Betty Trivell, Bob Plate, Marilyn Konzet, Kent Kleinman, John Beuscher, Joanne Kruszynski, Harvey Silverman, Louis Weisbord, Jeff Weisbord, Emilia Spoerri, Jennifer Linick, Paul Consiglio, Constance

Thanks to all who gave us permission to shoot at their location:
Patti Lein, Amagansett Eastside Tennis Club, Fleur and Leon Harlan, Lucia and Peter Gordon, Dunes Racquet Club

Dedication

I would like to dedicate this book to my mother, who has a big heart and a youthful outlook on life.

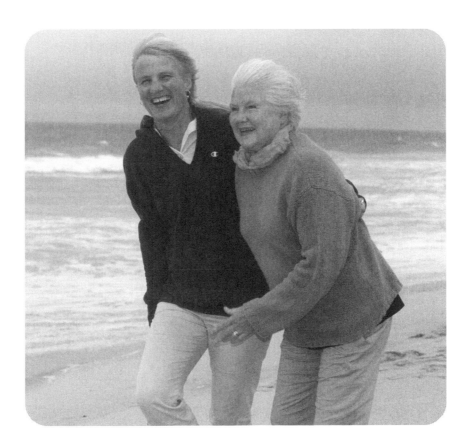

Contributors

Mike Bahel, Personal trainer, and owner of Body Tech Fitness Center, Amagansett, NY, e-mail: Body Tech@hamptons.com.

Bernard Brule, Private chef in Europe, New York City, and East Hampton, Long Island.

Gerald Curatola, D.D.S.: Director of The Center for Advanced Dentistry, East Hampton Dental Associates, P.C., East Hampton, New York.

Nancy DePietro, Licensed esthetician, certified aromatherapist and healing touch practitioner.

Vicky Magliaro, Licensed beautician, Owner Salon Fresca, East Hampton.

Miriam Novelle, Owner, Tea Salon and Emporium, New York, NY.

Susyn Reeve, Organization and Personal Development Consultant, Inter-Faith Minister, Sag Harbor, New York. e-mail: Susynr@aol.com

Jackie Storm, Ph.D., CNS, specializes in clinical and behavioral nutrition. Website: www.jackiestorm.com or via e-mail: jackiestorm@jackiestorm.com

Jane Umanoff, Prosperity Coach, Website: janeumanoff.com

Table of Contents

Introduction

To live long and look young, isn't that what we all want? We all know men and women who, no matter what their age, seem young; they have a certain glow, a vitality that is both beautiful and healthy. They exude confidence, and people are drawn to this confident energy. You can be one of those people; there are a few secrets that can help; but mostly simple truths. This book explores these secrets and truths.

The most important thing to realize is that beauty and health are not limited to surface appearances. While it is true that health is reflected in your posture, skin tone and energy level, true health and youthfulness are attitudes and feelings that radiate from the inside. Health is something we achieve in the way we live our lives; it involves our choices of activity, food and environment, as well as our attitudes and self-image.

It is very important to stay both physically and spiritually active, and to get in touch with our senses. For example, take a walk in a natural setting for at least one half-hour every day. This activates circulation and energy flow, and improves the condition of skin and hair. In addition, regular exercise can prevent many chronic diseases. Several scientific studies have found that moderate exercise, such as walking, lowers the risk of cardiovascular disease, cancer and other illnesses. Aerobic exercise and yoga relieve mental and emotional tension by helping to clear obsessive thoughts from our minds. Meditate or take the time to contemplate the world around you, sit still or lie down to a guided relaxation; this will revive your spirit

Once we are able to see the world as "our" world and ourselves as influential agents in the universe, we realize that we can continue to grow and learn at any age. It is never too late to try something new. If you have not been to an art exhibit, go to one. Or, plan a trip to a place that you have never visited before; it doesn't need to be far away. You may just want to explore a new neighborhood. Take that class you've always been meaning to sign up for. Stop procrastinating; if you make the effort to try something new, you will feel great! Continue to challenge yourself with new experiences, because once we get tight and inflexible in our mind and body, we age faster.

We all know the saying "you are what you eat." It is vital to provide your body with the nutrients it needs. As we get older, that may mean making a special effort to avoid preservatives and to make sure we get enough calcium in our diet. Eating a varied, balanced diet is important to rejuvenate the body. Don't eat the same foods all the time. That can become boring, and might lead to splurging on junk food. In our fast paced world, we don't always have the time to enjoy a meal at a leisurely pace, but it can be an invaluable part of your day. Set the table, light a candle and eat a meal with yourself, family or a friend. This setting will help you get more enjoyment from your meal. Try to eat at least one meal a day like this.

A clean environment with plenty of fresh air is important. It is great if you breathe clean, fresh air on a regular basis. Try to go to the seaside, or mountains, or to a nearby park. Natural sunlight also is essential. Try to get outside every day. If you need to be inside most of the day, try to work near a window. You also may consider purchasing special full spectrum light bulbs that simulate natural light for your workplace. If you live in the country, trees and plants probably surround you. If you live in a city apartment, buy some house plants or fresh flowers. All these factors will help to create a healthy, beautiful environment.

Design your home in a way that feels comfortable, relaxing and inviting. Take a look at what is and isn't working functionally in your home, and make appropriate changes. It might mean buying a certain kind of mattress or a new set of shelves; such small improvements make life easier yet cost very little. Color can affect your mood. Yellow often is very uplifting, blue soothing, and tans and reds nurturing. Take note of the colors that you like to be surrounded by and paint one room in your favorite color. If a room is painted white or a neutral color, hang a painting, poster or print that you enjoy.

To maximize your potential to stay healthy and young looking, you must also keep in mind the importance of balance in your life. When we are out of balance, we are more likely to be affected by stress. In Tibetan medicine, imbalance can lead to three types of stress: Wind stress, which includes muscle tightness; Stress of Bile, impatience and irritability, and Phlegm, which includes depression and fatigue.

Mind, body and spirit are intertwined. These three areas connect our physical, mental and emotional states. If we are out of balance, stress results and we feel tired, anxious or depressed. Many aspects of life can be out of balance. For example, if you work very long hours and take no time off to go to the gym, your body is in imbalance. The remedy can be to join a gym and go several times a week, practicing weight training three times, attending a stretch class one day, and getting a massage the next. Or, if you work a lot and spend no time on your personal relationships, the remedy can be to make a walking date with a friend once a week, get together for lunch, or give one another a foot massage.

I have studied and taught yoga for 25 years now. I started out as a modern dance student in New York City where I grew up amid a lot of distractions and without much exposure to nature. In my dance training, as in yoga, the focus was on breathing, centering, and leveraging and articulating joints. I have assimilated this information and passed it on to my yoga students. I continue to take yoga classes so I can learn and teach new techniques and postures. Yoga is the art of combining the awareness of the body, mind and soul. In yoga you work from the inside out; you notice how you feel and do what you need to do to feel more balanced. Since yoga is not a competitive activity, you improve by challenging yourself. It is important to take a class as often as you can with a teacher you really enjoy. While it is good to practice yoga alone, taking a class is necessary because the teacher can check your positions and make sure that you are not compensating. A good teacher encourages us to work through boundaries and habits that hold us back. I believe that the philosophy behind yoga can be applied to all things in life.

In this book I present things you can do to live long and look young whether you are in your thirties, forties, or eighties. You'll find suggestions on exercises, nutrition, massage and skin care. You'll also find sections on personal development and how to cultivate the vital spiritual and emotional components of good health and longevity. I hope you'll find the tips in this book inspiring and helpful as you continue your life's journey.

Lisa Trivell
East Hampton, 2001

Exercise

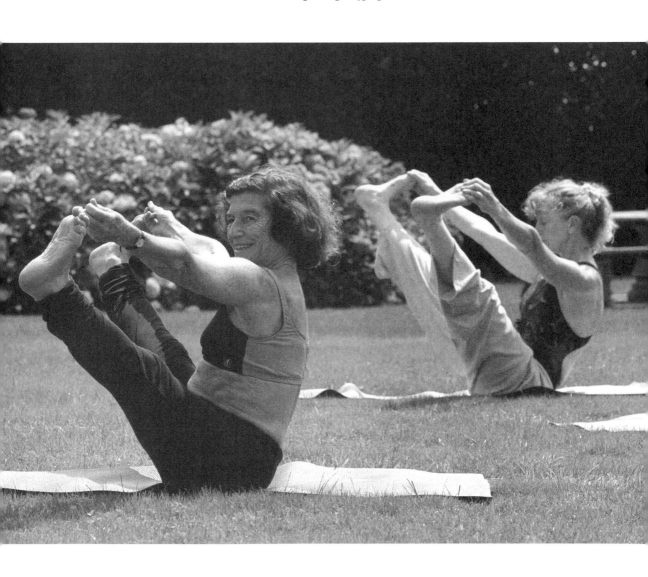

Live Long, Look Young!

Virtually nothing can make you feel younger or more alive than being physically fit. Exercise increases energy through the release of tension and endorphins. By concentrating on the activity you take your mind off of worries. In addition, it increases endurance and makes you stronger.

You don't need to take up huge chunks of time to get your exercise. When it comes to exercise, every minute counts. If you say you want to start to exercise, but don't have enough time or energy, you should think twice. The Surgeon General's Report on Physical Activity and Health (1996) found health benefits *from just 30 minutes of moderate activity* each day.

A report in the *Journal of the American Heart Association* noted that even 15 minute bouts of exercise—if done frequently enough—may be as beneficial as longer sessions. It is the total amount of time you spend exercising (with a goal of 30 minutes each day) not the length of each individual session that is important. Cross training is great too. You don't have to be a triathlete to cross train. Just alternate activities: for example, do aerobics one day, yoga the next. In general, you want to try to do some aerobics and yoga at least three times a week each.

The key is to find an activity that you truly enjoy and can do regularly. It doesn't make sense to depend on swimming if you don't have easy access to a pool, especially when it's cold outside. You also want to build exercise into your life so that it is convenient. Find a class or gym that is near your house or office. Some people can create their workout routines at home; others find they are more disciplined when they work out with a friend at the gym. Most everyone enjoys walking and it is convenient—it can be done anywhere. Try to go for a walk every evening after dinner. Don't feel guilty if something comes up and you have to miss your walk. Just resume the next day. Make sure you vary your routine so that you don't get bored.

When we work out we sometimes unconsciously favor certain muscles and don't stretch adequately. This causes tightness and may lead to injury. In this book, we introduce yoga and meditation, which increase flexibility, remind us to be in the moment and to use the full range of our muscles. We learn to increase circulation and work the body more efficiently. I believe you should incorporate yoga into your life, as you will see in the section on yoga in this chapter.

Before we go into some different exercise suggestions I first want to discuss an all-too-often neglected aspect of our physical lives: breathing.

Breathing

The breathing techniques and postures of yoga were developed many thousands of years ago and were prescribed to prevent disease because our breath is the most basic tool to purify and revitalize our bodies. In fact the way you breathe often is a reflection of how you think about yourself and how you relate to the world around you. If you breathe in a shallow way, you are not maximizing your potential as a person and all of your vital systems will function at a minimal level. However, if your breath is long and deep you are truly present in the world, allowing your respiratory system to function fully and completely. The way we breathe is a measure of our physical and emotional state. How fully and evenly we breathe is indicative of our level of stress. Breathing fully and correctly relieves tension and we end up with more energy available to us.

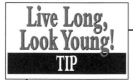

Smooth Flying

Simple breathing exercises can help eliminate anxiety. For example, if you get nervous flying on an airplane, particularly during take-off and landing, try the three-part breath: Fill your lungs with air as you inhale and hold for a few seconds, then slowly exhale completely. Repeat this exercise until you have flown through the turbulence or have landed. How well we feel is connected to how well we breathe.

Many of us need to re-learn how to breathe properly. This is easy because it feels comfortable. Try the following: Sit in a comfortable position, balancing your weight between your hips and crossing your legs. When you inhale, feel your lungs fill up three-dimensionally, like two balloons on a count of three. Feel the expansion to the front, sides and back (Be sure you don't suck in your stomach when you inhale). Fill up your entire lungs then slowly exhale on a count of three emptying them completely. Think of rejuvenating yourself with each inhale and releasing stress and tension with each exhale. You can practice this breathing technique in any stressful situation; for example, when you are stuck in traffic or having a stressful telephone conversation.

One type of breathing technique is the *Breath of Fire*. This technique strengthens your nervous system, cleanses your blood and expands the electromagnetic field of your body. The fire breath consists of taking short one-second breaths through your nose. As you do this, concentrate on pumping your breath out using your abdominal muscles. As you inhale, your abdomen should release; as you exhale, it should push in. Practice this breath 30-60 times and you will feel truly revived. This is good to do after guided relaxation or when you just wake up.

You can also use breath visualization as part of a guided relaxation or during meditation. Breath visualization uses the power of your imagination to unblock tension as the guided breath increases awareness and promotes circulation. There are infinite possibilities for visualizations, depending on your needs. Combinations include focusing on body parts, color and sound, as well as on mental, emotional and spiritual affirmations. On the following page an example of a **guided breath visualization** called "Breathe the Tension Away" is described.

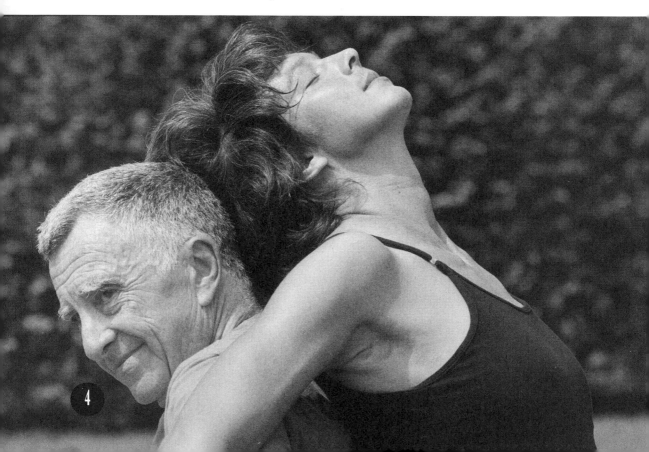

Breathe the Tension Away

Close your eyes, relax your body and release into gravity. Imagine your breath traveling to an area that is tight. Concentrate on sending your breath to that area. Take a full breath and on the exhale feel the tension leaving the area that is congested. On the inhale send circulation towards the tight spot; on the exhale feel the tension leave the area. Notice that you are starting to feel more relaxed.

Proper breathing oxygenates the blood—it increases the amount of oxygenated red blood cells and releases carbon dioxide as a waste. This sends more circulation to the entire body including, of course, the brain, which can stimulate your memory and creative processes. If you suffer from physical aches and tensions, try practicing full inhalations and long complete exhalations. As early as the fourth century B.C. the philosopher Chuang-tze said that men of great wisdom fetch their breath from deep inside and below, while ordinary men breathe from their larynx only. Even back then people were aware of the great value of deep respiration!

Here is an example of how full deep breathing is applied to yoga.

Sit down with your left leg straight out and your right leg bent. Move your right foot to the inside of your left leg. Interlace your fingers and reach up on the inhale. On the exhale, bend from the hip sockets and stretch over the left leg. Hold for a few seconds, inhale and stretch out further as you exhale. Repeat the breath three times. Feel the tightness in your muscles release with each exhale, as you stretch further. Do not bounce, but reach further with each exhale.

Another type of breathing is the *Kundalini breath.* For this breath you inhale through your nose and at the top of your breath you hold and lift your pelvic floor muscles. Start to feel the energy traveling up and down your spine. Exhale and release the pelvic floor muscles. Repeat the Kundalini breath several times until you become more aware of the energy traveling up and down your spine. On the inhale feel the energy traveling up your spine and on the exhale feel the energy traveling back down your spine. Establish a rhythm of breathing to help you balance the energy moving through your body.

Aerobics

Aerobic activities help to keep your body composition lean and your heart strong. Everyone should do 20-30 minutes of aerobic exercise at least three times each week.

Before we get into the different types of aerobic activities that you can do to look young, live long and feel great, I want to briefly say a few words about breathing and yoga and their relationship to aerobics. It is important to focus on proper breathing when doing aerobic exercise. This means taking the full diaphragmatic breaths that I talked about in the previous section in order to most efficiently circulate oxygen throughout your body, in particular to your working muscles. However, when doing aerobics you are breathing much faster than you would when doing yoga or meditating, so while you still inhale through your nose, you will exhale through your mouth during aerobic exercise. Do some yoga stretches before and after any aerobic activity. The stretches will help you to tune into your body, release tension, prevent injury and provide you with a sense of calm and well-being. Find an aerobic activity that you enjoy and is convenient to your location and schedule. This makes it easier to integrate into your life.

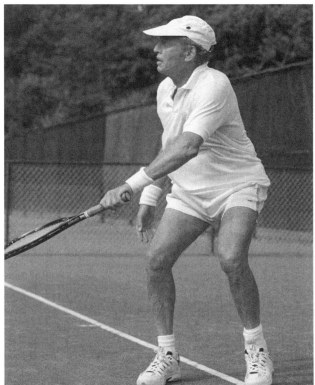

Walking

Going for a half-hour walk is a wonderful way to exercise and clear your mind of stressful thoughts. Take a walk alone or with a friend, around the block or in a park. It is particularly relaxing to walk by a body of water if you have the chance. Otherwise, simply find a neighborhood that you enjoy walking in. You might like a familiar route or try a brand new one and check out the scenery as you walk.

Focus your attention on the things that you pass. Notice the sights, sounds and smells around you. Awakening your senses helps you to relax and enjoy nature. If you are at the beach, take a sunset walk. If you are in the mountains, take a mid-afternoon hike. Or if you are in a city, take a walk to a museum and enjoy walking through an exhibition. This will stimulate your visual senses, take your mind off daily pressures and give you pleasure.

Walking tones and strengthens your body, and clears obsessive thoughts as you tune into your senses—the sights, smells and sounds. The rhythm of walking at a comfortable pace in itself is very soothing. Combine yoga breathing with walking for maximum benefit. They are two of the healthiest exercises you can do.

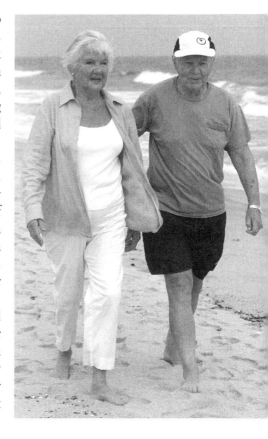

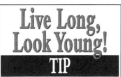

Walk and Talk

Instead of talking to a friend on the phone, get together and go for a walk. This way you'll see your friend, chat about what is going on and get a great aerobic workout all at the same time!

Biking

Biking is another wonderful aerobic exercise. Biking alone or with a friend is a great way to travel. Try biking to the library or grocery store instead of always jumping in your car. If you live in the country, try to find a bike path through the woods. If you live in the city, bike to work or in a park. You should make sure that you select a bike that is comfortable. Some people like mountain bikes and take off into the woods; others need a hybrid for travel on roads in cities and in the country; then of course, there are race bikes too. Whichever you select, make sure you wear a helmet for safety. You'll be surprised how fast the time goes as you take in the scenery on a relaxing ride!

Dance Class

So many dance exercise classes are offered today: jazz, low-impact aerobics, Latin, Ballroom or African dance—you name it and you'll probably find a class at a local gym or recreation center. Dance classes are a great way to release stress, learn something new (a key to staying young), have fun and get your exercise in all at the same time. Who doesn't like to move to music? Dance is one of the oldest forms of expression; it is liberating and makes us feel eminently youthful. Remember when you took your first dance class, or attended your first school dance? Recapture that feeling of freedom and emotional expression.

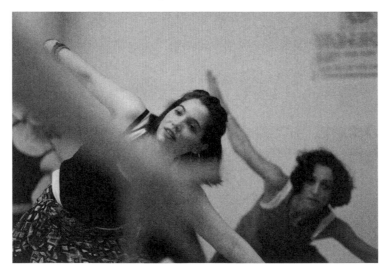

Water Exercises & Aquatics

Some people love the water. They like to live and walk by it and swim in it at every opportunity. These people naturally take to exercising in the water. But say you are a person who doesn't like swimming and getting your hair wet, you may surprise yourself by trying a water exercise class where your head is always above water.

Water is a wonderful medium to exercise in. You get so many positive results without straining your body. You feel light in the water because you are not fighting gravity. In the water, exercises that were extremely difficult are relatively effortless because the resistance of the water tones and shapes your body evenly. Water aerobics is a safe and effective way to increase strength and endurance. Working out in the water heightens your metabolism even when the workout is finished.

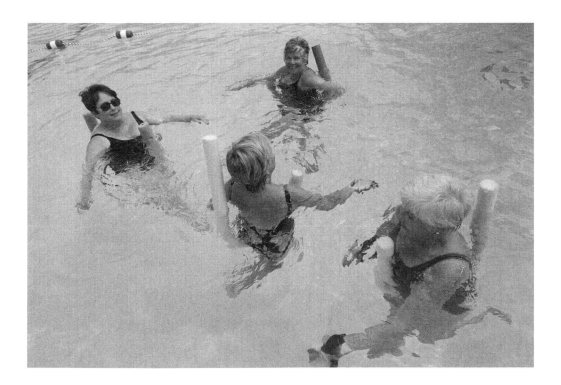

Live Long, Look Young!

Water workouts are beneficial to people of all ages and fitness levels. Water is a forgiving medium, reducing joint compression and the downward pull of gravity. Many participants who are unable to exercise on land can be very active in the water. The even pressure of the water helps to reduce swelling especially in the legs, ankles and feet. The water provides tactile feedback and improves sensory function in ways that are similar to the benefits in yoga. You start to move and feel areas of your body that may have been blocked. This gives you a great overall workout.

Most gyms and health clubs offer water classes, which are open to men and women of all ages and fitness levels. The classes are great social environments, where you can look forward to seeing friends. The many types of aquatic classes offered range from aerobics to body sculpting, stretching, toning or a combination. Other classes specialize in aerobics or exercises for people with limitations such as arthritis.

I offer classes in outdoor pools during the summer. It feels so great to be in the refreshing water with the warm sun on you, breathing in fresh air. The classes that I teach, like the workout I will show you here in the book, are well-rounded. We start with warm-ups. Many of the exercises are aqua yoga moves followed by an aerobic and spot toning section. I also will introduce aquatic equipment that enables you to jog, ski and bike in the water. You keep your hair dry and you can even keep your sunglasses on while working out. A piece of equipment called the noodle will help you remain buoyant. Webbed gloves can be worn to add resistance and strengthen your upper body during the workout. We wind down with a stretching segment, which draws upon yoga and emphasizes breathing and alignment. My aquatic students tell me that they feel relaxed after class but that they have more energy available to them throughout the day. This is a similar benefit of yoga.

In an aquatic class the water is kept at a comfortable 80-84 degrees so that your muscles can stretch properly and so you do not get chilled. The water is cool enough to regulate your body temperature. This way you are able to work out more vigorously during the aerobic section and not feel overheated.

The water is as an important element that connects the body, mind and spirit. You feel enlivened from being soothed by the water. It truly provides a holistic workout. Water exercises also increase sensation of muscles that you may not ordinarily use because you feel the water's resistance against your body. This greater awareness of moving a part of your body will carry over to everyday activities and the increased circulation and benefits will stay with you throughout the day. Try to take a class or do the workout featured below at least once a week.

The Aqua Workout

For all these exercises make sure you are in water that is deep enough to cover your chest. **Start out by performing each exercise five times and work up to ten repetitions. Repeat the following exercises on the both sides of your body unless it is a full body exercise.** Remember to breathe smoothly and fully throughout all the aquatic exercises.

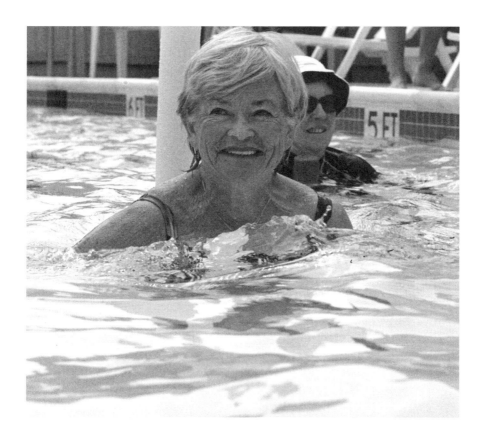

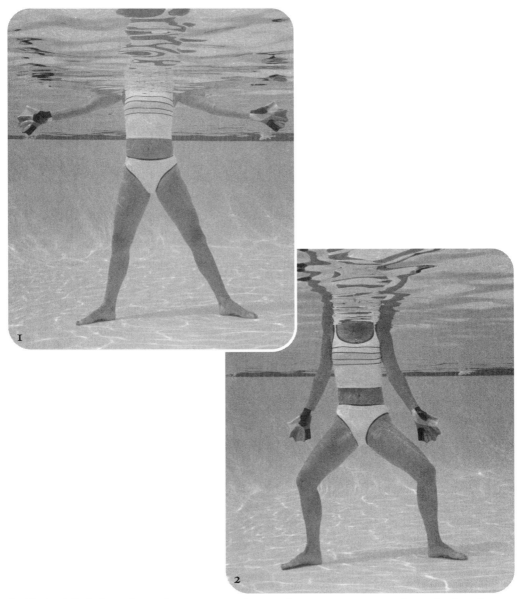

PLIES—With legs three feet apart and turned out, arms out to the side, bend your knees over your feet as you bring your arms into the center. *Benefits: tones your hips; great for strengthening your hip sockets and lower back.*

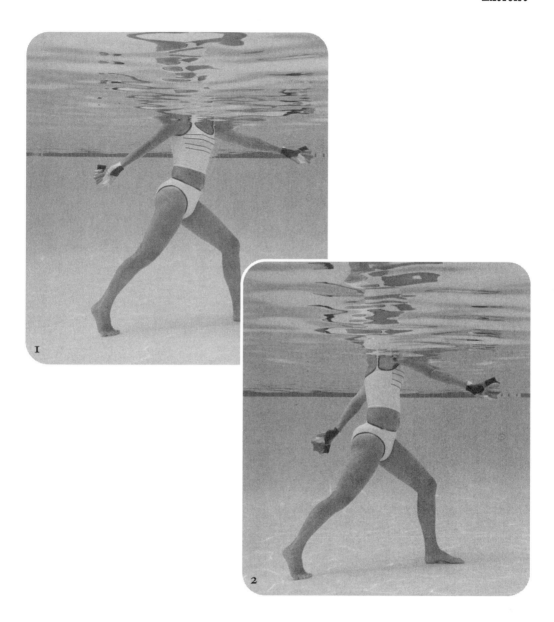

LUNGES—Moving your arms back and forth bend your front knee and straighten your back leg. *Benefits: warms up your hips and shoulders.*

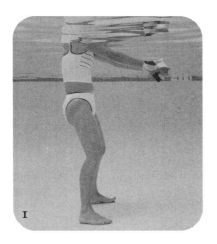 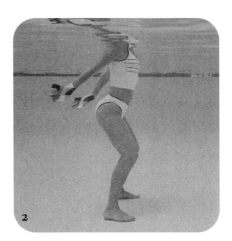

STANDING PELVIC TILTS—With your feet parallel, facing forward and knees slightly bent, tilt and arch your pelvis. *Benefits: relieves tension in your lower back and begins to activate your abdominals.*

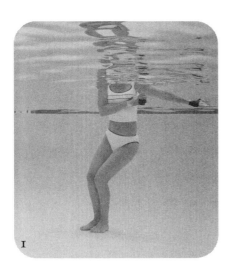 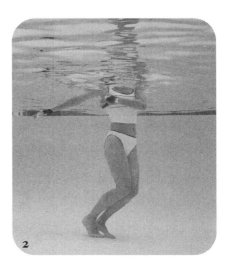

TWIST—Twist your hips and feet in one direction, your shoulders and arms in the opposite direction. *Benefits: awakens your waist muscles (obliques).*

The next three exercises, plus the noodle routine make a great 20-minute aerobic workout!

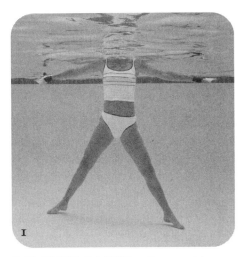 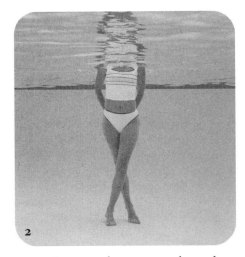

JUMPING JACKS—Start with arms and legs apart, jump and cross your legs, then jump and separate them. These can be done in place or across the pool. *Benefits: great for coordination and balance; integrates your whole body; improves circulation.*

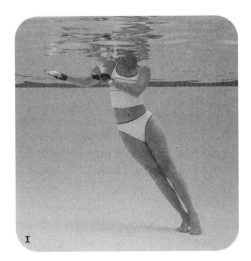 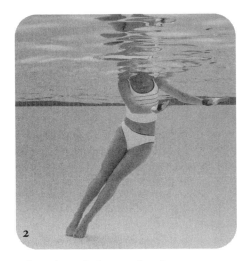

TUMMY TONER 1—Jump with your feet together from left to right, keeping your knees slightly bent. Imagine jumping over a barrel side to side. *Benefits: tones lower abdominals and obliques.*

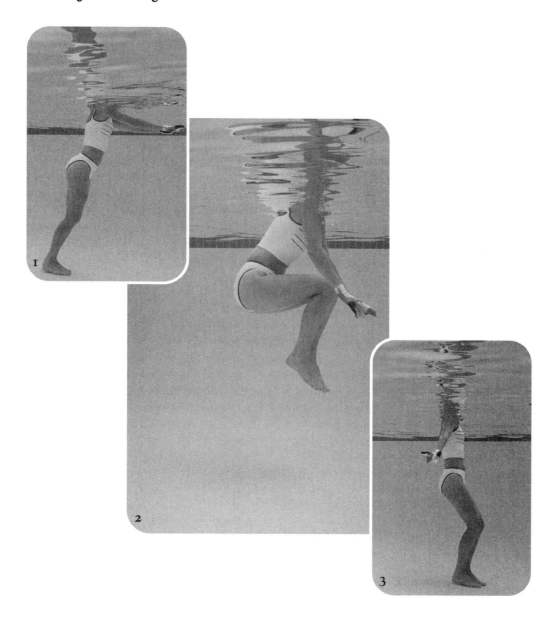

TUMMY TONER 2—Start with your feet together and your knees slightly bent. Jump forward and back, as if you are jumping over a barrel. *Benefits: tones lower abdominals.*

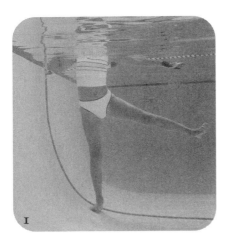 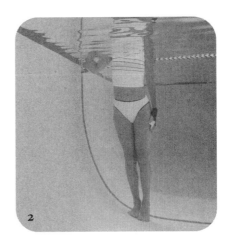

SIDE LEG KICKS #1—Kick your left leg to the side, knee facing forward, then bring it back to center. Your arm follows. *Benefits: firms your hips and love handles, and tones your outer thighs.*

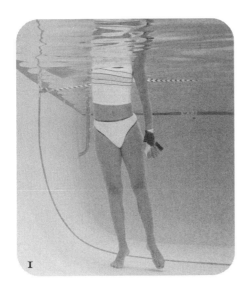 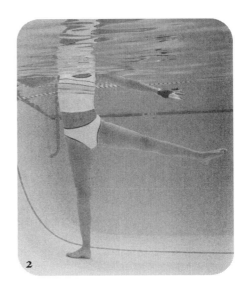

SIDE LEG KICKS #2—Turn your knee up and kick to the side. Your arm follows. *Benefits: works your quadriceps and hamstrings.*

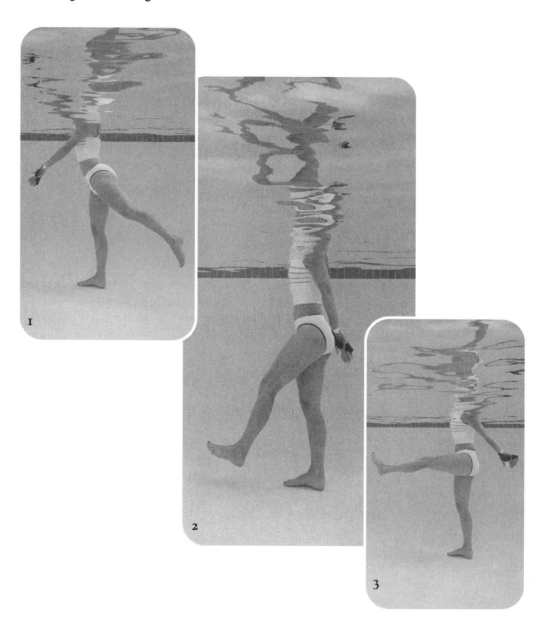

LEG SWING—Kick your leg forward, center and back, keeping it as straight as possible. Move your arms in opposition. *Benefits: great multi-muscle toner and stretcher.*

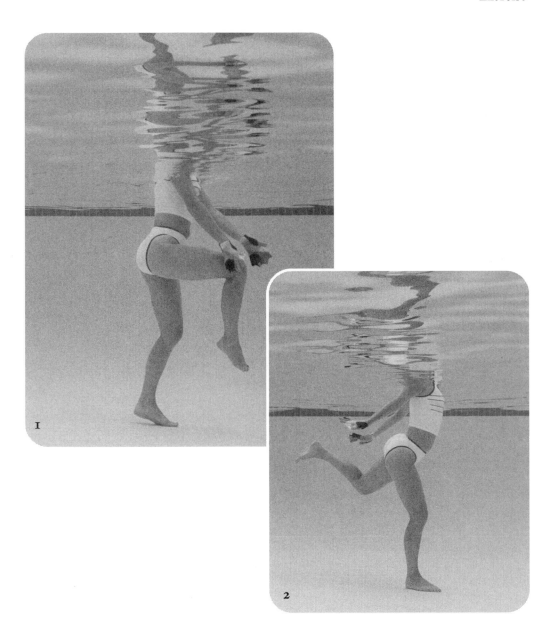

ROCKING HORSE—Rock forward and back, bending your knees. *Benefits: great overall toner.*

GET ON THE NOODLE

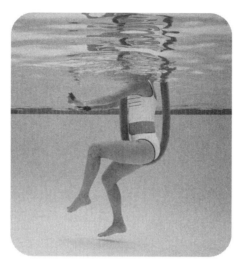

BICYCLE—Bicycle up and down the pool doing the breast stroke.

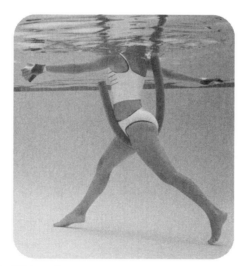

CROSS-COUNTRY SKIING—Move your arms and legs in opposition. Slice through the water to begin with your thumbs up and then press your palms down. Use your hands to increase resistance. Do this for up to five minutes for a great cardiovascular workout.

Yoga

At any age, yoga is a particularly wonderful form of exercise. It helps to maintain a strong spine and a supple body, releases tension and provides an inner calm. It is a very efficient form of exercise because within a yoga workout you tone and strengthen all the muscle groups in your body.

Yoga consists of breathing exercises and postures, which are done in different sequences to offer many benefits, particularly for the spinal column. Nerves that travel to all parts of the body and to all of our internal organs branch out from the spinal cord, which is located inside the bony vertebral column. When a vertebra is out of position, it affects the nerves and the muscles in the area as well as the internal organs related to those nerves. Muscular tension collects around the imbalanced area and can result in serious back pain. Yoga stretches the spine in all directions to release tension and keep the body in alignment. Doing this also helps to balance your nervous system. Yoga tones the muscles as well, so you attain full range of motion and an increased ability to contract and release. By practicing yoga, you get long, lean, toned muscles.

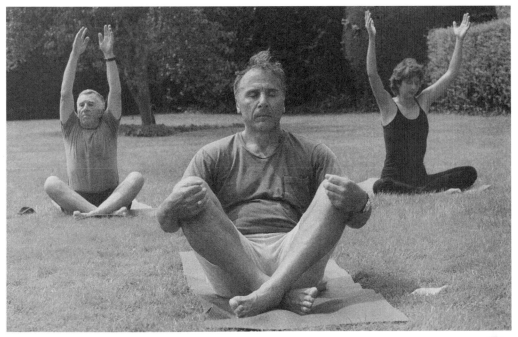

Live Long, Look Young!

Health and beauty are contingent upon the flexibility of our spines. When your spine is flexible and in alignment, the result is reflected in your whole body. A limber spine means a youthful body, while a stiff spine is an aging body. In yoga we strengthen the muscles that help us to sit and stand; this also helps us to feel more positive and look younger.

A routine of yoga helps to balance the spine by keeping two principles in mind. The first is to stretch the spine in all six possible directions: bending forward, backward, to each side and twisting to each side. This creates balance and symmetry in the spinal column. The second principle is that when you do an exercise that stretches the spine in one direction you should follow it with an exercise that stretches the spine in the other direction. For example, the plow, which rounds the spine is followed by the fish which arches the spine. Or, doing a seated spinal twist in one direction is followed by a spinal twist in the opposite direction.

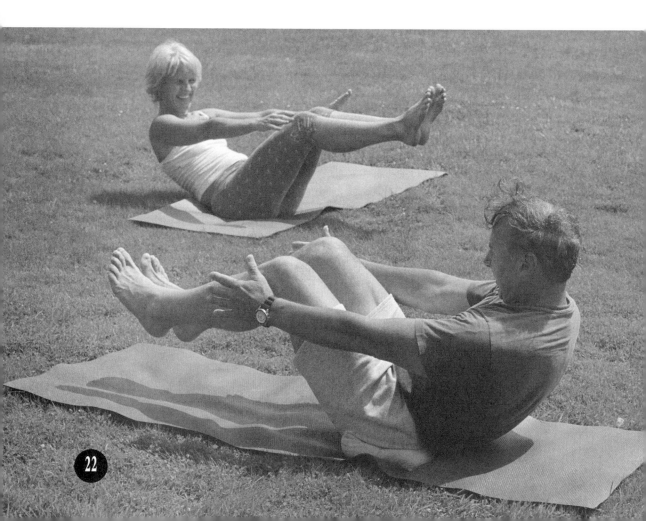

In yoga it is very important to take the time to consciously breathe through the nose in an unbroken rhythm. To breathe is our most natural instinct, but one that we have forgotten to perform properly. When we are babies we breathe most naturally, through our diaphragm. The stomach rises on the inhale and lowers on the exhale. Yoga involves breathing consciously and rhythmically throughout the poses. When you are practicing yoga, you are tuning into yourself. You awaken your senses. By your senses, I mean all the senses your body—hearing, smell, taste, touch, sight and the sixth sense—intuition.

Finally, yoga helps you to become more kinesthetically aware, improves posture and heightens the sensory functioning of the body. It helps you to bring into the light areas that might have been in darkness or numb. Once you are more attuned to feeling a place in your body, you move it more freely and without tension. You end up with more energy and less stress.

Acuyoga

Great sages practiced yoga, as a system of breathing and postures, over 6000 years ago. At about the same time, acupressure was developed. Acupressure is the science behind the channels of energy that travel through our bodies. These channels of energy are formed by synapses in our nerve endings; they travel through pathways that go through muscles, tendons and organs. When we combine acupressure with yoga (acuyoga) we stretch, tone and balance the meridians, receiving many benefits for our organs and hormones. Why? When you stretch a meridian it releases energy. Daily practice of acuyoga promotes longevity.

Many people feel that through their practice of yoga and meditation, their intuition becomes stronger. It is good to get signals from your intuition throughout the day. In a world where we often over-analyze situations, we need at times to look inward for the answer. It is important to acknowledge the higher self inside and outside us. Prayer or meditation can lead to peace, love and creativity, which encourage harmony and happiness. More on the spiritual aspect to being healthy and staying young appears later in this book.

The Yoga Workout

Remember to breathe through your nose throughout the yoga workout and to hold each stretch for three breaths.

Seated Yoga Positions

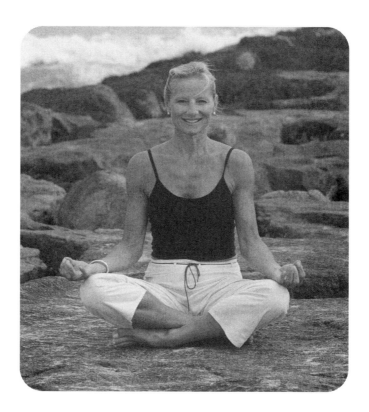

SEATED CROSS-LEGGED POSE—Sit in a comfortable position with your legs crossed in front of you. Resting on your sit bones, drop your shoulders and lift your stomach, chest and head. Take full breaths in and out of your nose, counting to three as you inhale and exhale. *Benefit: warms up hip sockets, encourages correct breathing, and improves posture.*

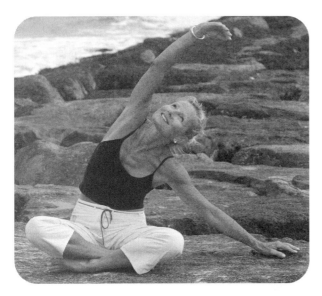

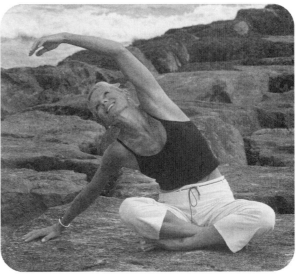

SEATED SIDE STRETCH—Sit in the basic cross-legged position, with your sit bones planted on the ground. Place your left hand on the floor, then stretch your right arm over your head and stretch. Return to center and repeat with your opposite arm. Perform three times on each side. *Benefit: tones stomach and torso muscles, and stretches the back.*

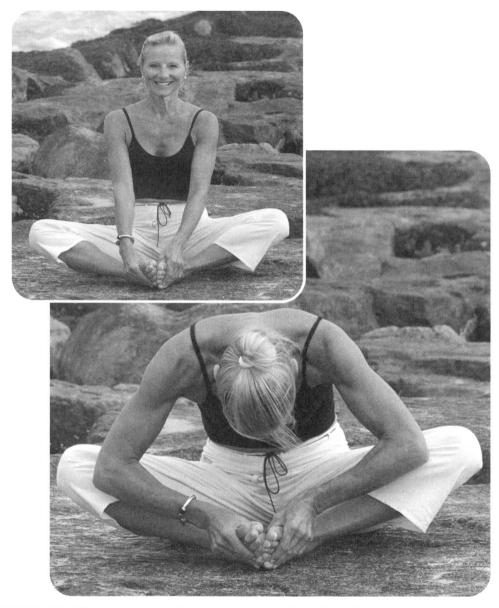

BUTTERFLY—Sit on your hip sockets with the soles of your feet together, your pinky toes touching, and your knees out to the side; stretch your head down to your toes. *Benefit: opens hip sockets, and releases lower back inner thighs, and sacrum.*

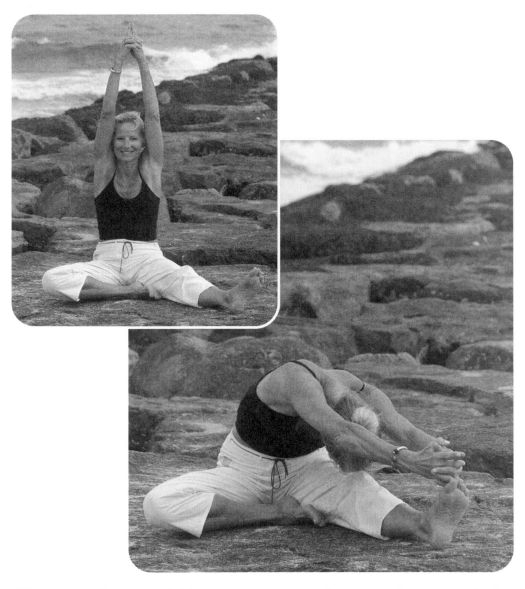

HURDLER—Bring your left leg into your right thigh and straighten your right leg. Exhale as you stretch towards your straightened leg, and inhale as you return. Hold your position, take three full breaths, and repeat on other side. *Benefit: prevents sciatica and limbers up the ankles, knees and hip sockets.*

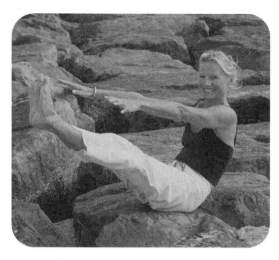

BOAT—Balance on your sit bones and straighten your legs as much as possible. Hold your arms out in front of you for balance. Hold for a count of 10 and repeat. *Benefit: tones your stomach muscles*.

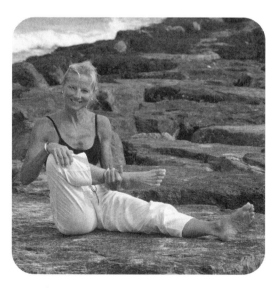

ROCK THE BABY—Balance on your sit bones, with your legs stretched out in front of you. Keep one leg straight; bend the other and cradle it to your chest. Rock from the hip. Switch sides. *Benefit: stretches the hip sockets*.

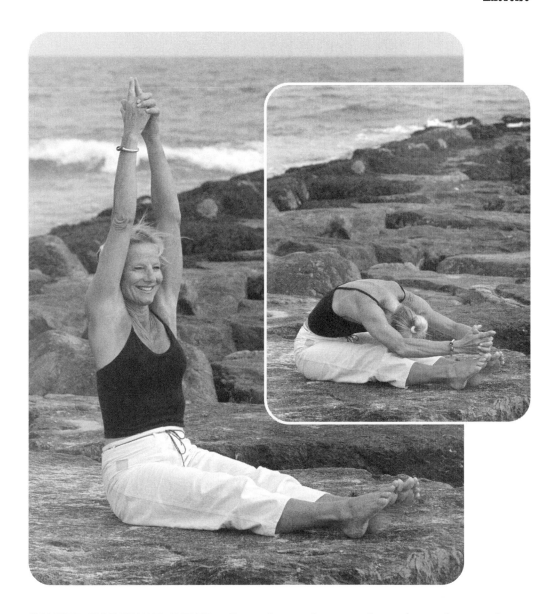

SEATED FORWARD BEND—Sit with your legs straight in front of you and your arms up. Inhale. Exhale and stretch your arms and torso towards your toes. Hold. (You can bend your knees slightly if you are tight.) *Benefit: stretches the lower back and the back of your legs.*

Standing Yoga Positions

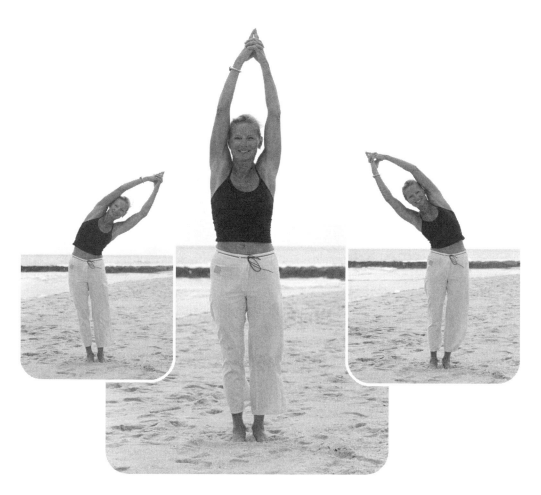

HALF MOON—Stand with your feet together or slightly apart if it is easier to balance, interlace your fingers, point your index fingers, and reach up to the sky. Inhale as you reach up and exhale as you press your arms to the right, your hips to the left. Hold and breathe. Return to center. Then reach your arms to the left and your hips to the right. Take a full breath. Repeat twice on each side. *Benefit: increases energy, strengthens the muscles in your torso and back, and increases flexibility in the spine, correcting bad posture.*

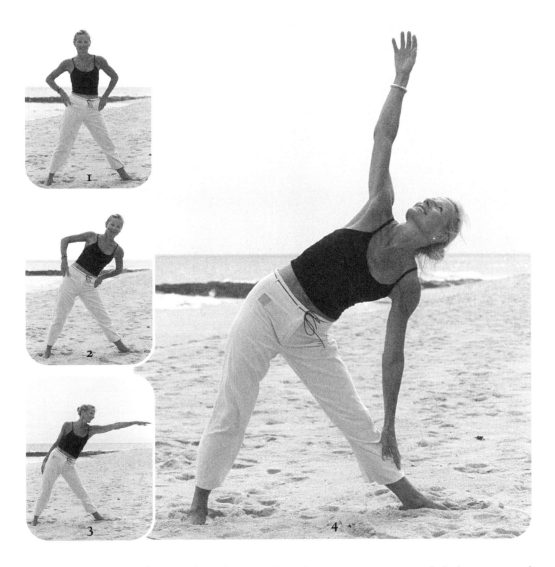

TRIANGLE—With your feet three to four feet apart, turn your left foot out and line up your left heel with your right ankle. Place your arms by your hips or stretched out to the side, parallel to the floor. Then, tilt back from your tailbone, moving your entire back and not just your waist. Slide your left hand down your left shin and stretch your right arm up above you. Reverse. *Benefit: tones the waist, hips, thighs, and backs of legs, and promotes balance.*

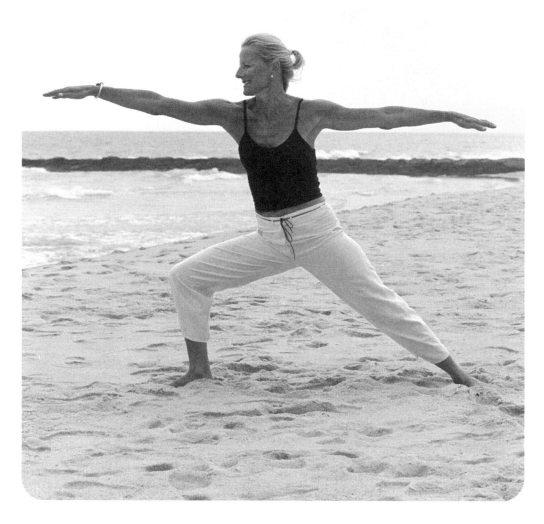

WARRIOR—From the Triangle Pose, bend your knee over your foot while keeping your thigh parallel to the ground. Keeping your palms down, lift your arms out to the side and look out towards the tips of your fingers. Hold the pose for 10 counts and repeat on other side. *Benefit: strengthens legs and helps align the back.*

SALUTATION

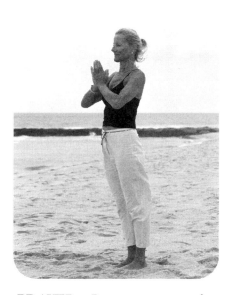

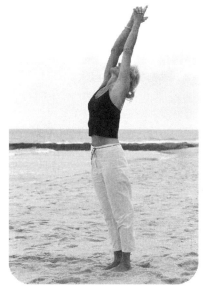

1. **PRAYER**—Bring your palms together in the middle of your chest along your sternum.

2. **HALF MOON BACK BEND**—Bring your palms together above your head, pointing your index fingers. Arch your back and lift our chest.

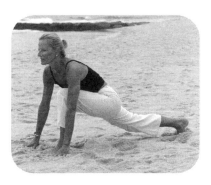

3. **LUNGE RIGHT LEG BACK**—Drop your right foot approximately four feet behind you. Keep your left knee bent over your toes and lengthen your neck. Focus on a point on the ground ahead of you as you lift your stomach muscles.

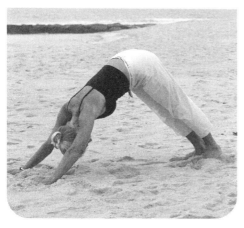

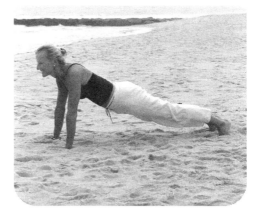

4. **DOWN DOG**—Bring your left foot behind you. Press your hands and feet into the floor and lift your hips high in the air.

5. **PLANK**—Bring your body parallel to the ground. Tighten your butt and abdominal muscles as you stretch your arms out straight. Lengthen your back.

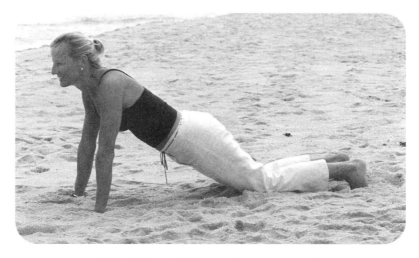

6. **PLANK VARIATION**—From the plank pose drop down to your knees, chest and chin.

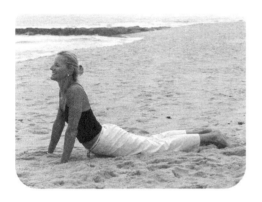

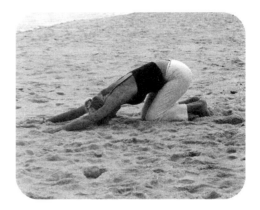

7. **UP DOG**—Slowly bend your elbows and swing your hips forward to your hands, with your knees and feet on the ground.

8. **CHILD POSE**—Release your pelvis and drop your butt to your heels. Stretch your arms out in front of you and lower your head to the ground.

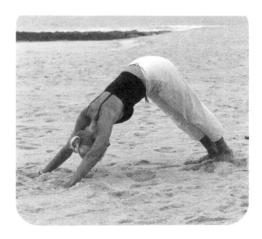

9. DOWN DOG

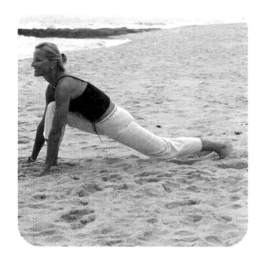

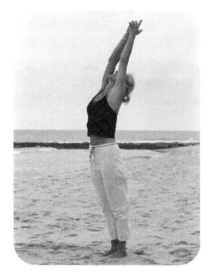

10. **LUNGE LEFT LEG BACK—**
(Same as p.33, only this time bring your left leg behind you.)

11. **ROLL UP TO HALF MOON BACK BEND**

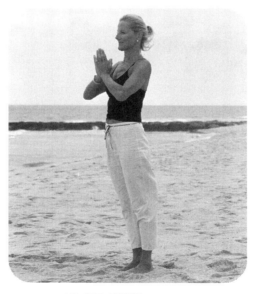

12. **PRAYER**

Ground Yoga Positions

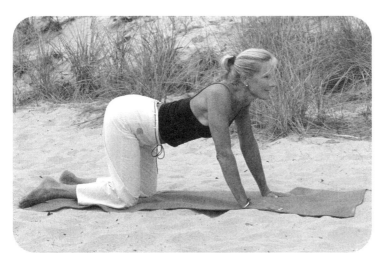

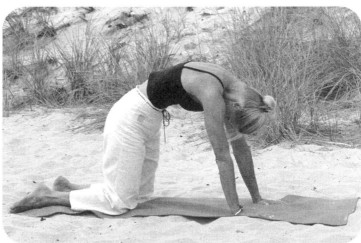

CAT—On your hands and knees, with your hands under shoulders and your knees under your hips, arch and round your spine. Inhale as you arch, exhale as you round. Repeat 10 times. Move slowly and concentrate. *Benefit: lengthens the back, and warms the muscles spine, and digestive organs.*

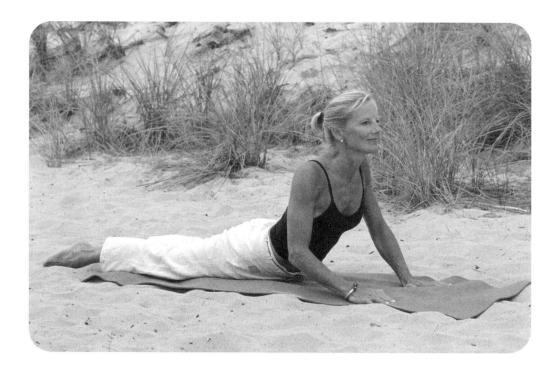

COBRA—Lie on your stomach with your hands directly under your shoulders. Breathe in and then exhale as you lift your head, upper back and stomach. Keep your hips on the ground and your elbows by your side. Breathe. Slowly release your chin as you relax back into the floor. *Benefit: strengthens the upper and lower back, and stimulates internal organs.*

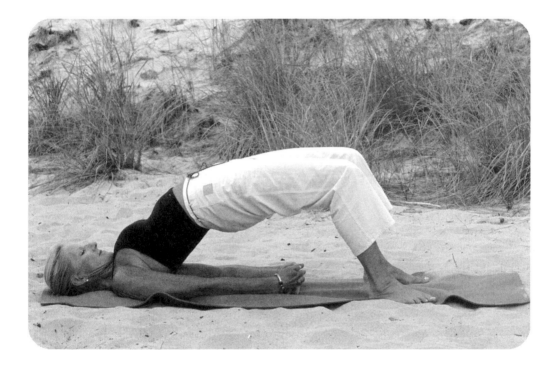

HALF BRIDGE—Start with a pelvic tilt and roll up vertebrae by vertebrae all the way up to the shoulders. *Benefit: balances your nervous system, strengthens hips, and releases tension in the neck and shoulders.*

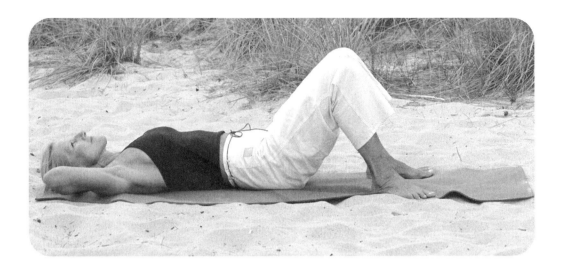

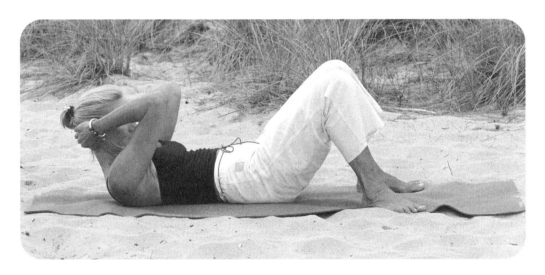

YOGA SIT-UP—Begin with your back on the ground, your knees bent and your hands behind your head. Cradle your head with your hands and exhale as you lift your head and upper body. *Benefit: tones stomach muscles.*

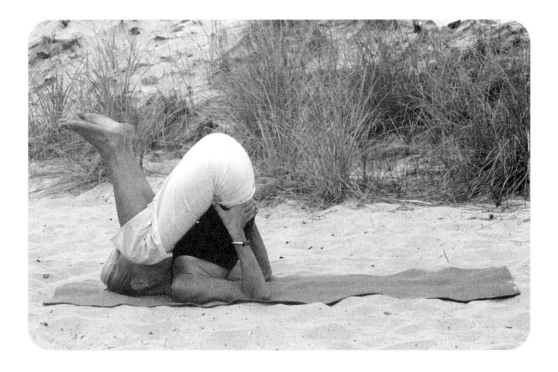

PLOW—From a seated position, slowly roll your legs up over your head reaching your toes toward the floor behind you. Bend your knees towards your shoulders and release. Clasp your arms under you or support your back. *Benefit: conditions the nervous and endocrine systems.*

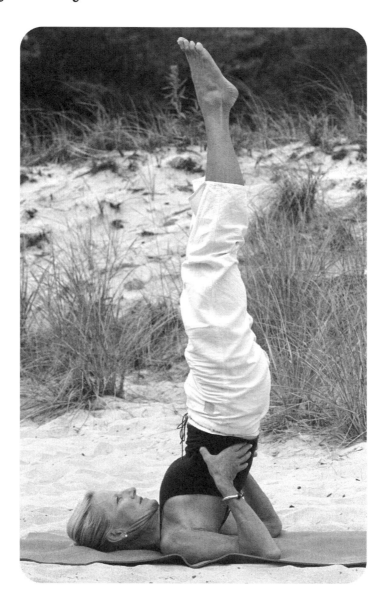

SHOULDER STAND—From the plow position, slowly raise your legs up towards the ceiling as you support your back. Hold for one to three minutes. Be careful not to rotate your head. *Benefit: reverses circulation and releases excess tension in the neck.*

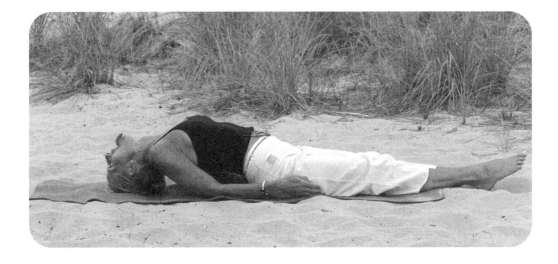

FISH—Lie on your back, bringing your feet and legs together and relax. Lift your body up on your elbows and arch your back from your tailbone to your neck. Work on releasing weight from your elbows, and stick out your tongue. Hold. *Benefit: balances the back and nerves after doing shoulder stands and tones the chin.*

Modified Seated Yoga Poses

Do these at your desk or while traveling. Remember to breathe fully.

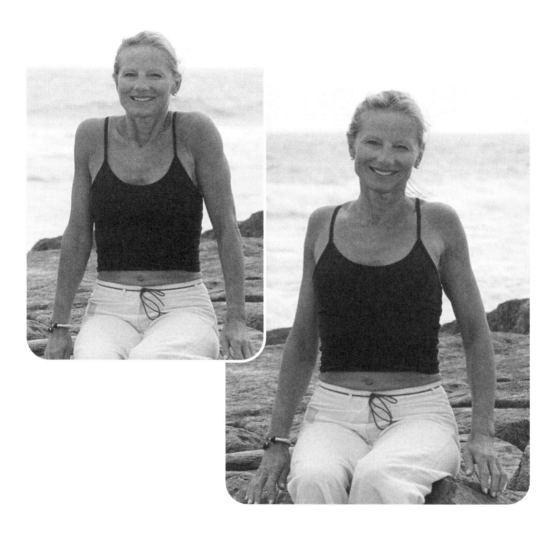

SHOULDER ROLLS—Roll your shoulders up, back, and around three times in each direction. *Benefit: releases shoulder tension and improves posture.*

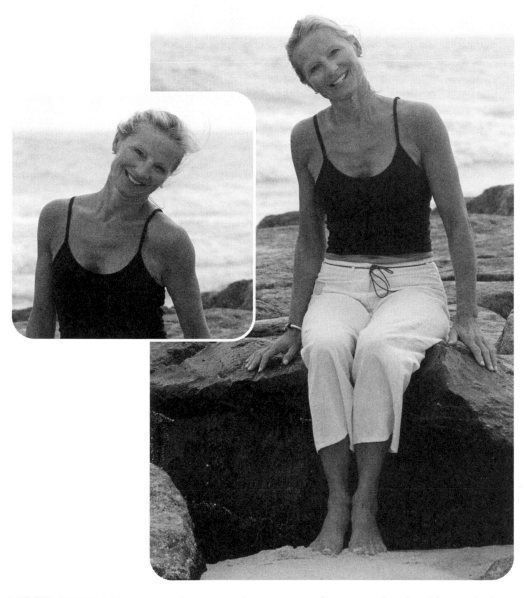

NECK STRETCH—Stretch your right ear towards your right shoulder and then your left ear towards your left shoulder. *Benefit: releases tension in your neck and increases circulation to the brain.*

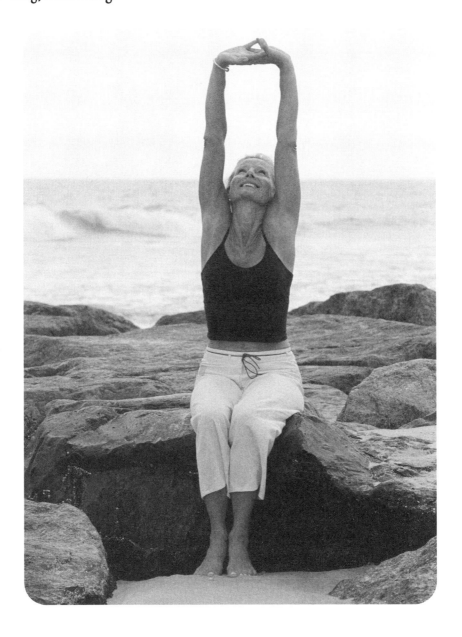

STRETCH UP—Interlace your fingers, palms to the sky, and stretch up. *Benefit: stretches the shoulders and releases tension in the neck and shoulders.*

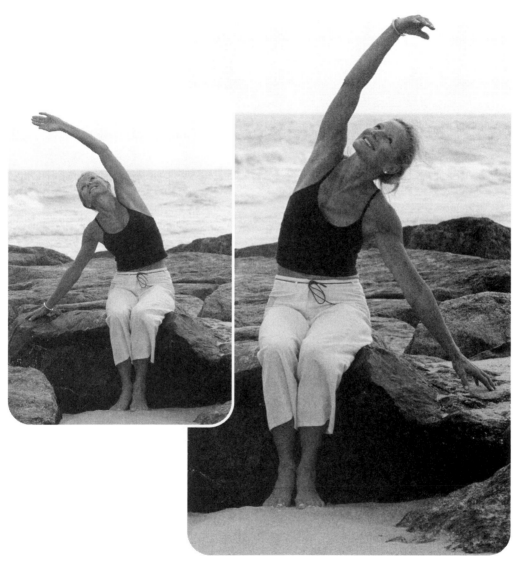

SIDE STRETCH—Sit in the basic cross-legged position with your sit bones planted on the floor. Place your left hand on the floor and stretch your right arm over your head close to your ear. Return to center and repeat on other side. Perform three times on each side. *Benefit: tones the stomach and torso muscles, and stretches the back.*

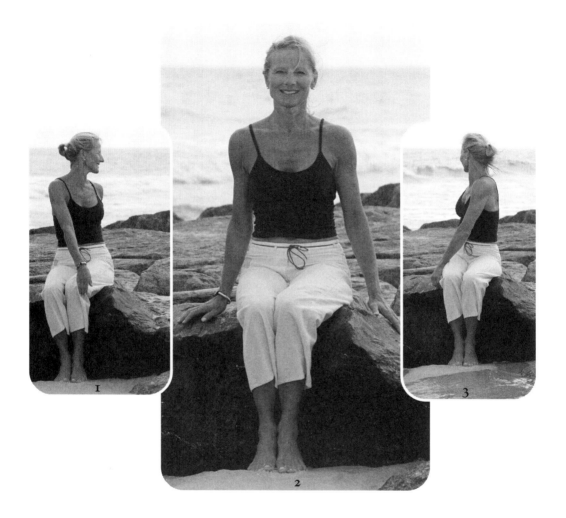

SPINAL TWIST—Rest on your sit bones with both legs in front of you. Bend your right leg over your left leg as your reach your right arm behind you and your left arm against the outside of your right thigh. Twist from your pelvis through your lower, middle and upper back. Twist, lift and breathe before gently releasing to the left. Repeat on your other side. *Benefit: rejuvenates the nervous system and increases flexibility in the spine.*

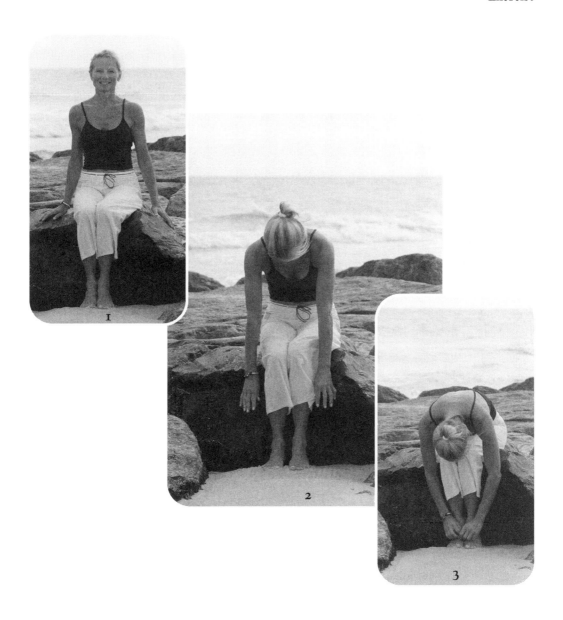

ROLL DOWN, ROLL UP—This is similar to a forward bend, but done from a seated position. Roll down headfirst and roll up head last. *Benefit: balances muscles on both sides of the spine.*

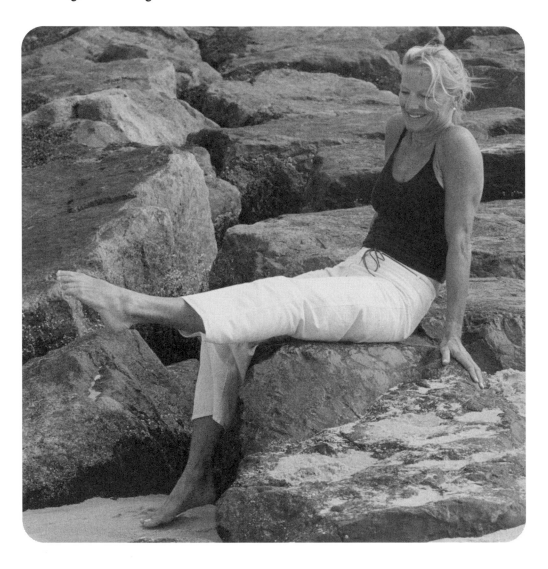

ROTATE ANKLES—Point and flex your foot, then rotate in a circle. *Benefit: strengthens ankles and prevents swelling.*

Weight Training

Training with weights helps to develop and define muscles, keeps your bones strong and your body toned as it combats the effects of gravity.

Weight trainer Mike Bahel (see profile) likes to think of training the body as a whole. He believes that while you need to isolate muscles at times you should balance your workouts so that you work your whole body. He recommends working out at the gym or at home with weights and dynabands two to three times a week. Mike suggests doing ten to fifteen reps of each exercise. When you plateau—after about five weeks of training—increase the weight gradually until you are at a level that you want to maintain. After that, you can try a different exercise instead of increasing the weight to challenge your muscles. For example, if you have been doing leg extensions, do squats or lunges to work some of the same muscle groups.

Before you start to weight train, warm up aerobically for about ten minutes to prevent injury. Always start weight training from the ground up. Begin with exercises for your legs, then back, chest, shoulders, biceps and triceps. In a sense you are working your larger, stronger muscles first.

There are two phases to each exercise: the concentric phase in which the muscle shortens, and the eccentric phase in which the muscle lengthens. For example, when doing a bicep curl, the concentric phase is when you bend your arm as you raise the weight, and the eccentric phase is when you extend your arm as you lower the weight. The stretch comes from the eccentric part of the movement and this is where you are getting most of the strengthening benefit. Mike recommends performing each exercise on a three-three count, shortening to three counts then lengthening to three counts.

As in yoga, your stomach muscles are the keys to stabilizing your back. It is very important to strengthen the center of your body. Learning yoga and applying it to strength training is extremely beneficial because it strengthens the core of your body (torso). In addition, the breathing awareness you get from yoga is extremely helpful in weight training. Remember to exhale as you exert, inhale as you lengthen.

Being able to focus on the muscles you are working is the key to weight training. A warm-up of yoga exercises before weight training or taking a yoga class in between your weight training days will increase your ability to isolate muscles because in yoga you are continually increasing sensory awareness of different muscle groups. Also, in both yoga and weight training, you are thinking three-dimensionally—not only about the front of the body, but also the side and the back. A great example of this is the deltoid (shoulder) muscle group. There are the anterior (front), medial (middle) and posterior (rear) deltoid muscles. An effective workout tones all of these.

Working with dynabands and free weights is very convenient. You do not have to go out and buy expensive gym equipment. Simply invest in some free weights and two dynabands of different resistance and you'll be on your way to a leaner, more toned you.

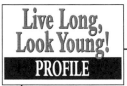

Mike Bahel—34 Years Young—Personal Trainer

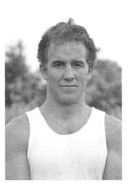

The average age of Mike's clients is between thirty four and sixty five, with a 60/40 ratio of women to men. "I love working with the thirty to forty year age group because that is when health issues of aging start to take place," he says. Through training his clients and teaching them how to exercise efficiently, they strengthen their muscles as well as their immune systems.

"A committed exercise program done several times a week plays a key role to living a healthier, stronger and longer life. Other factors are also important such as eating healthy and avoiding drugs, smoking, alcohol, pollution and stress," he says. Mike notes that it is never to late to start a fitness routine and at any stage, it gives you so many benefits. "With the increasing risks of heart disease, breast and colon cancer, and osteoporosis, an exercise and diet plan will play a major preventive role," Mike says. "For instance, women after menopause have an increased risk of osteoporosis; with a resistance training program they can reduce or eliminate their chances of contracting this condition.

Mike specializes in combining resistance strength training with cardiovascular and flexibility exercises. A graduate from Loch University in Pennsylvania with a B.S. in Recreational Fitness Management, Mike is studying fitness and active living for seniors and the effects of aging. He is certified with the American Council on Exercise and the Senior Fitness Association.

He recommends yoga for clients who have some arthritis, bone loss or acute joint pain. "Yoga has very little impact on the joints. It offers a safe, effective way to isolate the muscles and connective tissue for strengthening and flexibility," Mike says. In addition, he recommends doing some yoga before or after weight training.

During our interview, Mike and I agreed that yoga's greatest contributions to training are that it really teaches you how to concentrate on proper breathing and on how to isolate the different muscles groups. By learning how to isolate a specific muscle, you learn how to use it in a specific exercise. You want to engage all the muscle groups in your individual fitness program and yoga helps you to get in touch with areas you may have been avoiding. If you do not use certain areas of your body, tension can gather there and the muscles lose shape. According to Mike, the best ways to relieve tension are yoga, massage, exercise, meditation and physical activity.

Mike says his secret to staying young is to wake up every morning and make a promise to take part in some activity that he finds enjoyable or rewarding. "Whether it's riding a bike, lifting weights, swimming, doing yoga, rollerblading, walking in the park, playing tennis, jumping rope or throwing a frisbee, commit twenty to thirty minutes or more to it a day. If you have trouble finding that much time at once, then do it in ten minute bouts. The key is active living," he says. "Instead of driving to the store, walk or bike there; instead of using an escalator, use the stairs."

Eating healthy foods by following the food pyramid guidelines and cutting out saturated fats also will lead you to a longer, healthier life. But Mike acknowledges that it may not always be possible to eat the healthiest foods.

"Everyone is entitled to a snack, slice of pizza or a hamburger. Try to be smart and sensible. Don't overeat or overdo it. If you have something not so healthy to eat, it's not the end of the world. Just eat something healthy at your next meal. Moderation and sensibility are the keys to a healthy diet," he says.

Free Weight Workout

You'll need a bench and two pairs of free weights for this workout, one heavier than the other. Perform ten to fifteen reps of each exercise, and one to two sets. Exhale on the exertion.

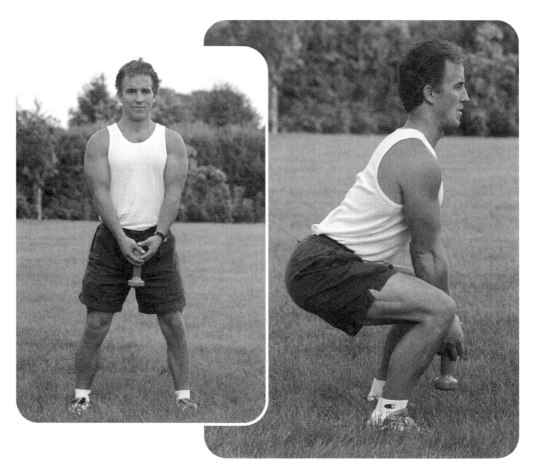

SQUAT—Stand with your legs shoulder width apart. Hold a weight with both hands. With your knees in line with your toes lower and lift your body, keeping the natural curve in your back. Make sure you keep your chest over your thighs and that your knees do not go past your toes. Squat to 90 degrees. This works your quads, gluteals and hamstrings.

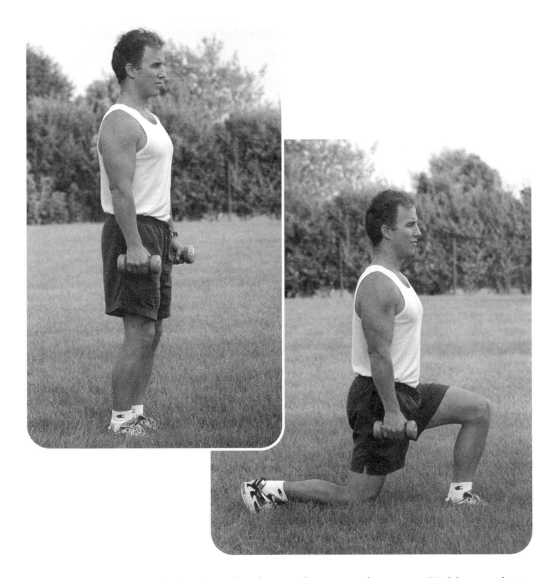

ALTERNATE LUNGES—Stand with your feet six inches apart. Hold a weight in each hand. Step forward with one leg, keeping both feet facing front. Bend both legs so that the rear leg almost touches the floor and the front leg is at ninety degrees. Hold the stretch. Then push off back to the starting position. Repeat on each leg. This works the quads, gluteals and hamstrings.

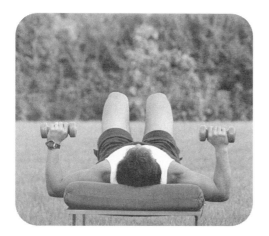 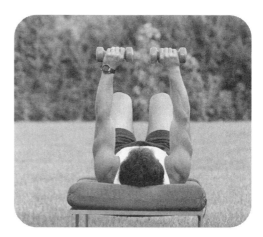

CHEST PRESS—Lie on your back on a bench or the floor, with your arms bent at ninety degrees, perpendicular to your chest. Press the weights up over your chest bringing them slightly together until your arms are straight. This works the pectoral muscles of your chest.

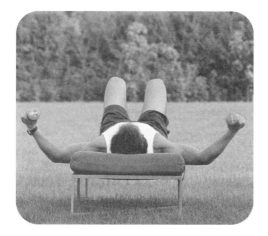 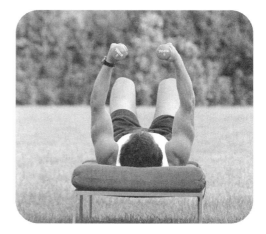

CHEST FLY—Lie on your back with your arms out to your side (palms up) and slightly bent. Bring the weights together as you squeeze your chest. Finish with your hands six inches apart. This works your pectoral muscles.

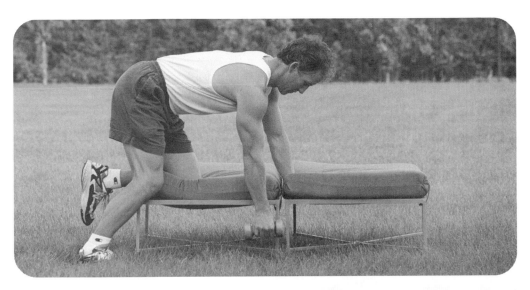

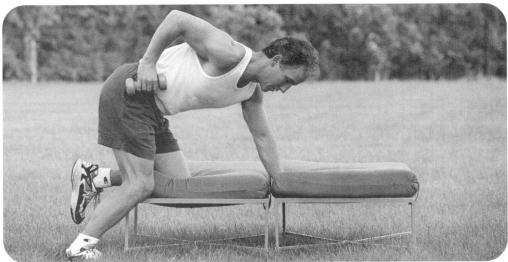

BENT OVER ROW—Kneel with one knee on the bench. Place one hand on the bench. Keep the arm with the weight straight. Bend at your elbow, bringing the weight up towards your ribs. Pull from your back. This strengthens your back.

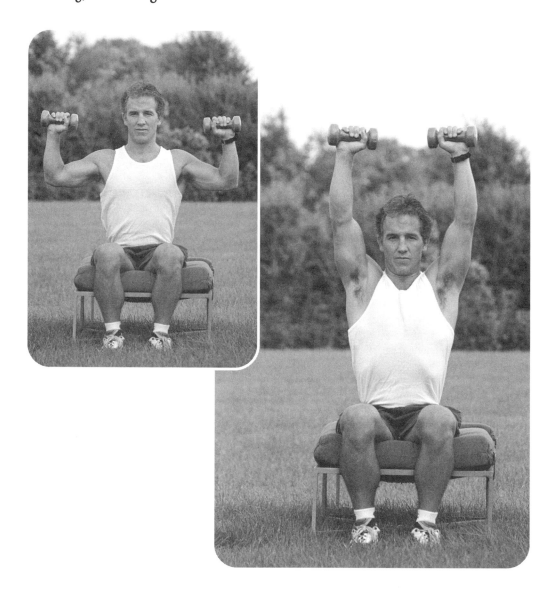

SEATED OVERHEAD PRESS—Sit with your arms out to the side and bent at ninety degrees, palms facing front. Press the weights overhead bringing your hands in slightly. Finish with your hands directly over your shoulders. Keep your back straight. This tones your shoulders.

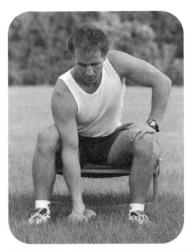 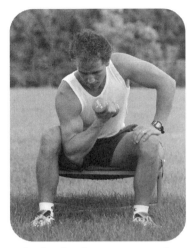

SEATED CONCENTRATION CURL—Sit and rest the back of one arm against your inner thigh. Curl that arm up towards your shoulder, squeezing your bicep as you curl. This tones your biceps.

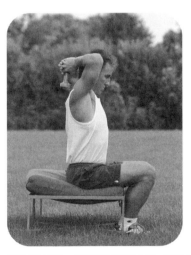 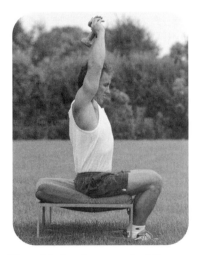

SEATED OVERHEAD TRICEP EXTENSION—Sit with both arms holding a dumbbell above your head, your arms fully extended. Lower the dumbbell, bending from the elbows so that the dumbbell is behind your neck. Your arms should be bent at ninety degrees. Press the dumbbell back up over your head with your arms fully extended. This receives the triceps.

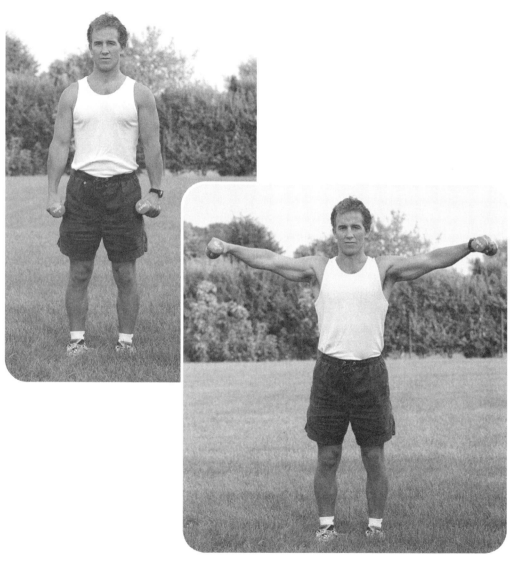

LATERAL RAISES—Standing straight feet parallel. Both arms down to the side, palms down. On exhale, lift the arms to become parallel to the ground.

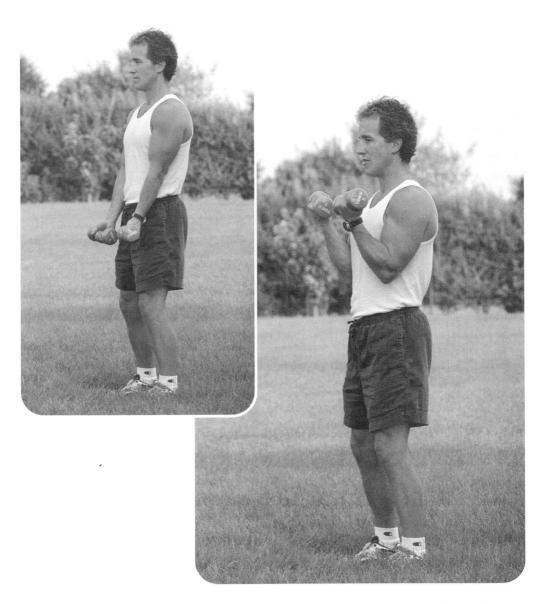

BICEP CURL—With a weight in each hand, alternate bending and straightening each arm at the elbow. This works the biceps.

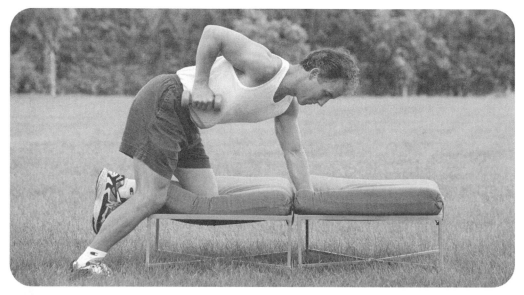

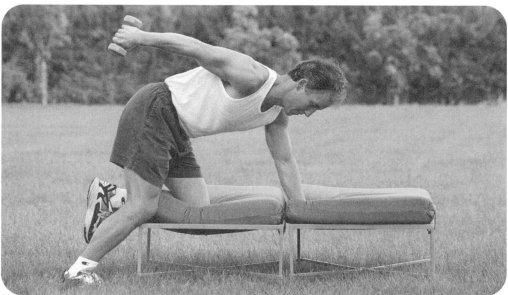

TRICEPS EXTENSION—Lean on a bench, keep your back straight. With a weight in your free hand, bend and straighten your elbow. Repeat on the other side. This works the triceps.

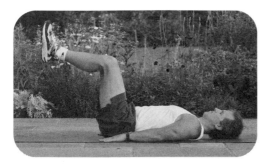 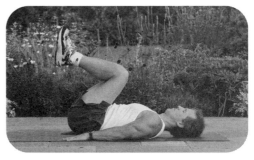

REVERSE CRUNCH—Lie on your back, with your hands at your sides and your legs up (knees bent at ninety degree). Tilt your pelvis forward. Pull your knees in towards your chest, lifting slightly while you contract your abdominals.

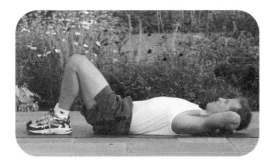 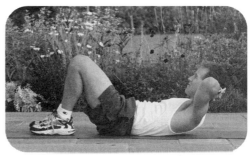

CRUNCH

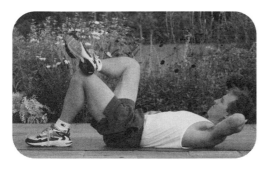 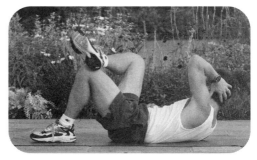

OBLIQUE

Dynabands

Dynabands provide a portable workout that is both a fabulous weight resistance routine and very efficient. To do this workout, you'll need dynabands of different resistances and a bench or chair. Start working out from the feet up, always leaving the abdominals for last in order to keep the center of your body strong and supportive through the workout. The general count on the exercises is three as you contract three as you lengthen. Remember that the lengthening is as important as the shortening so you need to pay full attention to this part of every exercise. Repeat each exercise ten to fifteen times and perform one or two sets. Go to the point of exhausting the muscle. Be consistent. If you start out with one set of fifteen reps for an exercise, carry that through the entire workout. Breathe evenly and fully. Inhale as you lengthen, exhale as you contract. This is where an awareness of yoga breathing can be applied to weight training. If you only have time for a fast workout, do not speed up the exercise. Instead, do just one set of fifteen reps instead of two. Support yourself with your stomach muscles.

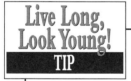

Take Your Workout on the Road

With a dynaband, you can literally take your workout anywhere. Whether you are travelling for vacation or business, a dynaband provides a wonderful and convenient source of resistance for muscular training.

The Dynaband Workout

Perform 10-15 reps of each exercise. You may do either one or two sets.

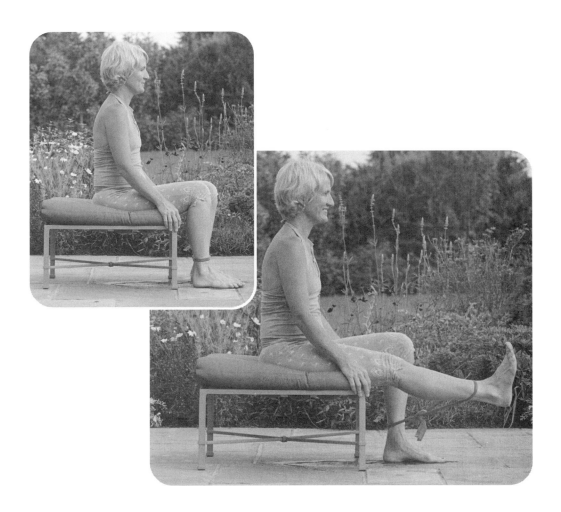

LEG EXTENSION—Sit down with the band around your ankle. With your back straight (less than ninety degrees), raise and extend your leg from the knees, keeping your toes up. Repeat exercise on each leg. This tones the quadriceps.

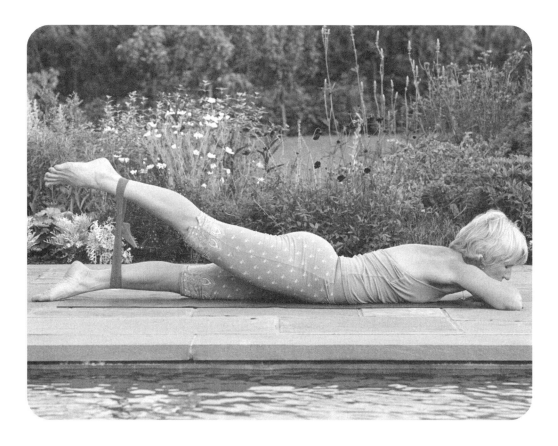

GLUTEALS—Lie on your stomach, with your legs together. Raise one leg up toward the sky, keeping your knee locked. Repeat exercise on each leg.

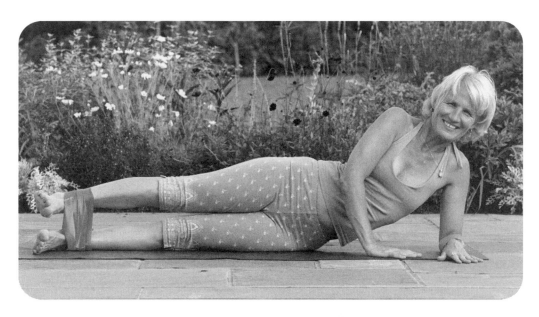

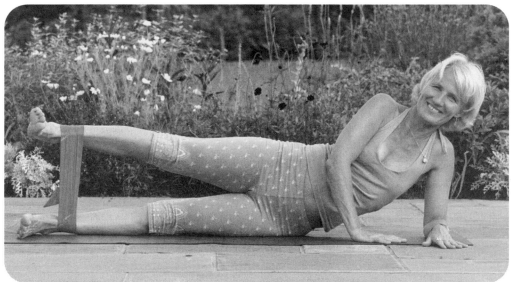

ABDUCTORS—Lie on your side with your legs two inches apart and lift your top leg, keeping your legs straight. Repeat exercise on other side.

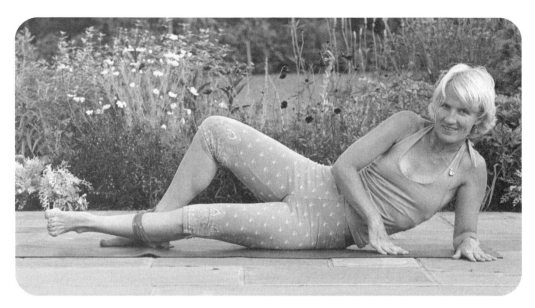

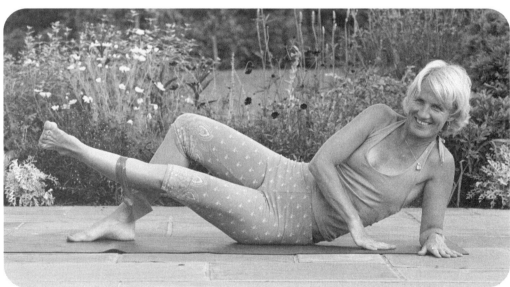

ADDUCTORS—Lie on your side and bend your top leg at the knee, placing your foot behind your lower leg. Raise your bottom leg, keeping it straight. Repeat on other side.

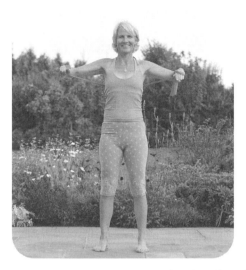 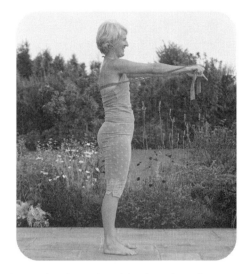

CHEST PRESS—Wrap the dynaband around your back at shoulder level with your elbows flexed at a ninety-degree angle. Think about your pectoral muscles as you press forward.

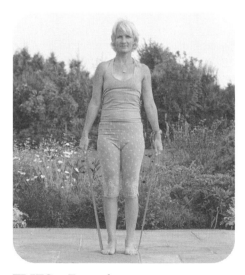 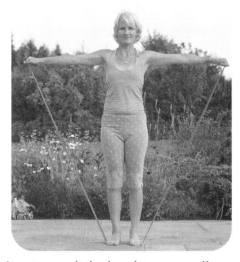

FLIES—Extend your arms out to your side, keeping a slight bend in your elbow. Press your hands together isolating the chest. Inhale as you separate your arms and exhale as you bring them closer together.

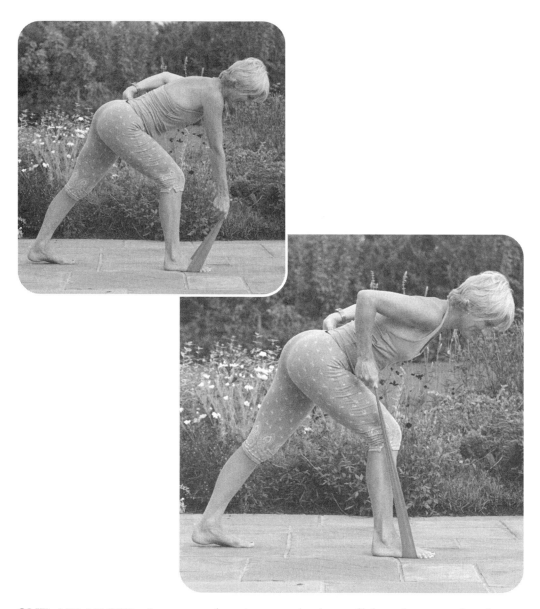

ONE ARM ROW—Lean over, keeping your back parallel to the ground and your arm straight. Pull the band up towards your ribs, bending your elbow to ninety degrees. Pull from your back.

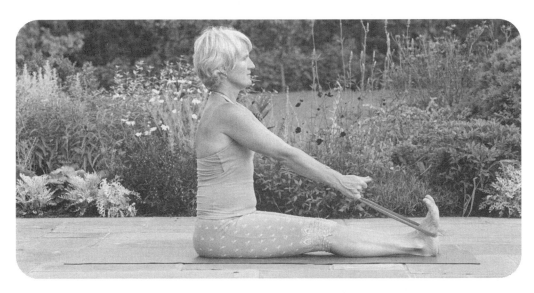

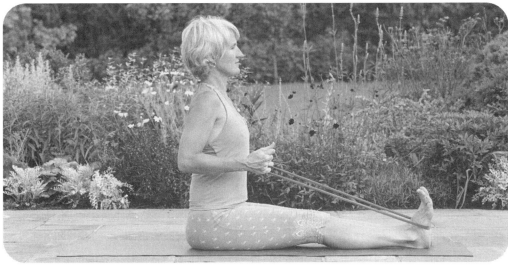

ROWS—Sit on the floor with your back straight and your arms extended out in front. Pull your elbows back past your sides, making sure you pull from your back. Squeeze your shoulder blades together at the finish.

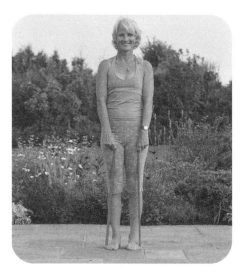 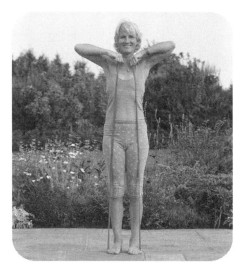

UPRIGHT ROW—Start with your hands down in front of your thighs. Pull the bands up towards your shoulders, keeping your elbows up and pointed out. Pull from your shoulders.

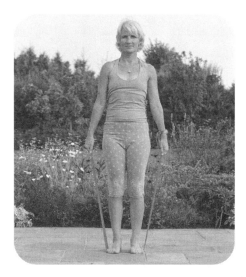 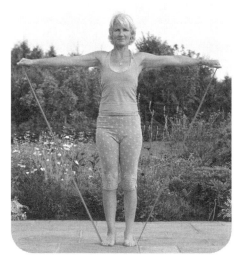

SIDE LATERAL RAISE—Start with your hands down next to your hips. Lift your arms out to the side to shoulder height. Keep your arms straight.

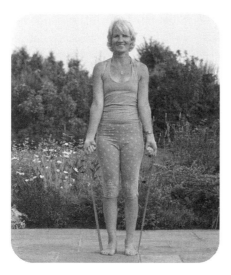 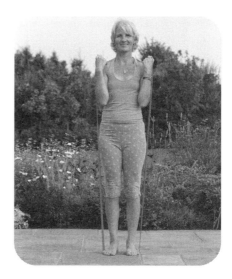

BICEPS CURL—Start with your hands down at your sides, palms out. Pull the bands up towards your shoulders, bending your elbows.

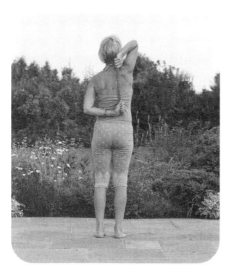 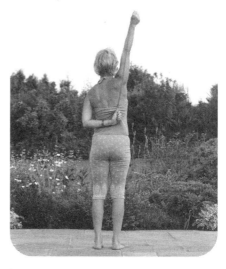

ONE ARM OVERHEAD EXTENSION—Hold one end of a band behind your lower back, the other behind your neck. Extend your hand overhead, straightening your elbow. Extend from the triceps muscles at the back of your arms.

Osteoporosis

Bones go through a constant state of loss and re-growth. As a person ages, there is more loss than growth. This can lead to a condition called osteoporosis, when the bones become thin and fragile, and break easily. Osteoporosis can be especially threatening to women at or beyond menopause, when your body starts to produce less estrogen, the hormone that protects against bone loss.

The first signs of osteoporosis are seen in the spongy bone of the spine, hip and wrist. After about the age of thirty five, bone is broken down faster then it is made. A small amount of bone loss after thirty five in both men and women is normal. Too much bone loss can result in osteoporosis.

Research shows that watching your diet and doing regular exercise, including the weight-bearing type, can prevent osteoporosis and in some cases increase bone mass. Just as muscles become stronger with exercise, so do bones. You should do a combination of weight-bearing exercises, such as walking, tennis, weight training and yoga exercises. Women should be sure to take in enough calcium through diet and supplements. In her book *Exercises for Osteoporosis* (Hatherleigh Press 2000), Dianne Daniels provides a variety of programs to treat and protect against osteoporosis (see resource section in appendix).

Symptoms of osteoporosis do not usually occur until there is considerable bone loss so it is important to take preventative measures. A few symptoms are back pain or tenderness, loss of height, and slight curving of the upper back. Consult your physician and be tested for osteoporosis if you think you may be at risk. Testing can help both women and men can reduce the risk of becoming frail and fracturing their hip or spine later in life.

The sections in this book on dynabands, weight lifting and water exercise present you with wonderful ways to help prevent osteoporosis.

Facial Exercise

Your face is the presentation of your self to the world. Exercises can bring back or maintain a natural glow and vitality.

We speak in this book of reaching and toning all the muscles in the body. It is important to include facial exercise as well. By practicing facial exercises at the end of your yoga routine or at any time during the day, you awaken your face. These exercises tone the underlining structure of your face and increase blood circulation to the skin. The result is a firmly toned face with a healthy looking complexion. By toning and stretching your facial muscles, you can maintain or regain a young looking face.

When you do facial exercises you release excess tension in your face. In my massage and yoga practice, I come across many people who have tension in their jaw muscles. This can lead to headaches and sometimes even migraines. Other people grind their teeth, especially at night, which can lead to premature dental work.

Practicing a regular facial workout will help you to maintain a relaxed, younger, healthier and vital-looking face. As we age, some faces start to look pale. They flatten and elongate. Due to lack of use and gravity, faces sag. Some people's faces get frozen into the same expressions that can cause or deepen wrinkles in the face. You may notice people who hold a lot of tension in their faces. They are either always squinting or have a perpetual fake smile or frown.

Notice how refreshing it is to look at and communicate with people whose faces are expressive! The face is what is presented to the world first. When we are in a state of tension, it often appears first on our face, freezing any expression. We want to be relaxed enough so that we can look and communicate freely and with expression. Your face can become a map of your habits well as a reflection of your emotional history and state of mind.

While plastic surgery deals with the symptoms of an aging face, facial exercises deal with some of the causes. You need to practice the following exercises regularly to see and feel the results. First try doing the facial routine on its own. Then, add it onto a yoga workout twice a week. You also can practice facial exercises interspersed throughout the day. Try some while you are at your desk, on the computer, on the phone or in the shower. You can continually improve your appearance, release stress and let go of fixed expressions.

We are willing to spend hours toning the muscles of the body through different forms of exercise. Why not add a facial exercise routine that will only take minutes?

The Facial Workout

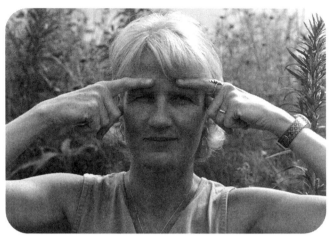

FOREHEAD LIFT—Place your index fingers about one-half inch above your eyebrows. While your fingers are pressing down, concentrate on lifting your eyebrows. Do these mini-lifts twenty times. Then, hold your eyebrows up for twenty counts.

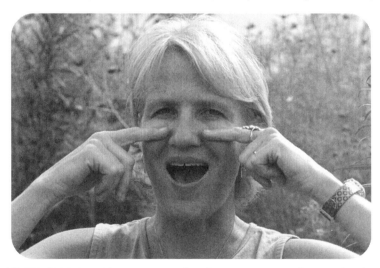

CHEEK DEVELOPER—Place your index fingers on top of your cheeks. Open your mouth and form an "O"; hold the "O" shape, keeping the upper lip pressed against the teeth. Now smile with the corners of your mouth and release. Repeat twenty times.

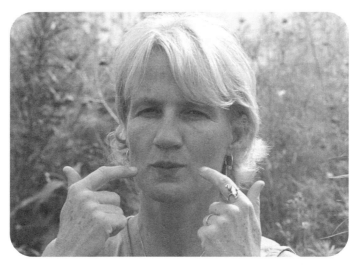

LIP SHAPER—Press your lips flat against your teeth, then lift the corners of your mouth up and down. Do twenty times.

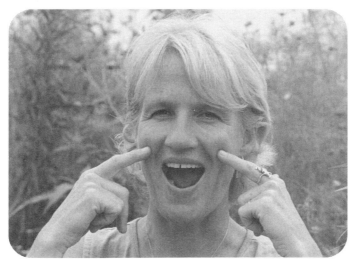

WRINKLE ERASER—Place your index fingers lightly on your cheeks. Open your mouth into a big "O" shape then back into a smaller "O" shape. Do ten times.

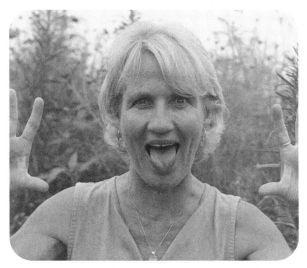

LION—Stick your tongue out as far as you can. Hold (This is great to prevent or correct double chin.)

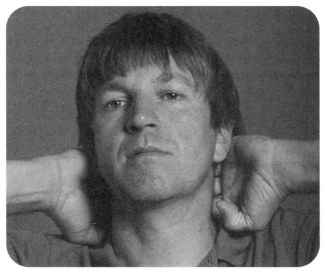

HEAD ROLLS—Roll your head from the top of your neck, making a small circle three times in one direction, then three times in the other direction.

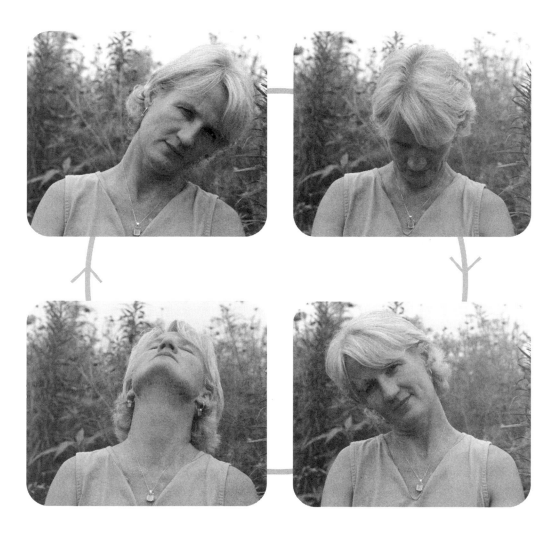

NECK ROLLS—Roll your neck slowly from the seventh cervical three times in one direction, then three times slowly in the other direction.

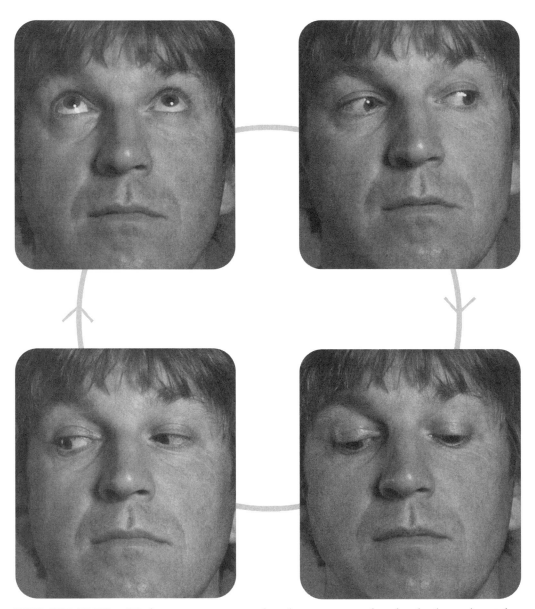

EYE CIRCLES—Without moving your head, gaze up to the sky, look to the right, look down, look to the left. Make three smooth circles to the right, moving through any areas that are tense. Close your eyes. Open and reverse the exercise.

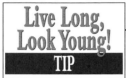

Find Your True Age

Functional age is measured by the ability of an individual to be totally active and agile. *Chronological* age refers to a person's age measured in years. Many adults have advanced chronological age, but young functional age, helping them feel young throughout their lives.

The American Medical Association Committee on Aging found it almost impossible to distinguish between the effects of aging and the effects of inactivity. This is why it is so important to do some exercise everyday, such as yoga in the morning, complimented by a weight lifting routine.

The following is a list of some conditions associated with aging that can be prevented by exercise:

- Low energy
- Obesity
- Arthritis
- Weakness\poor muscle strength
- Stress\hypertension
- High cholesterol
- Constipation
- Back problems
- Insomnia

- Senility
- Heart condition
- Depression
- Chronic pain
- Decreased lung capacity
- Stiffness
- Osteoporosis
- Diabetes
- Bad posture

Many of these conditions can be improved or alleviated by regular physical exercise. Research shows that exercise initiated at any age will provide many physical and psychological benefits.

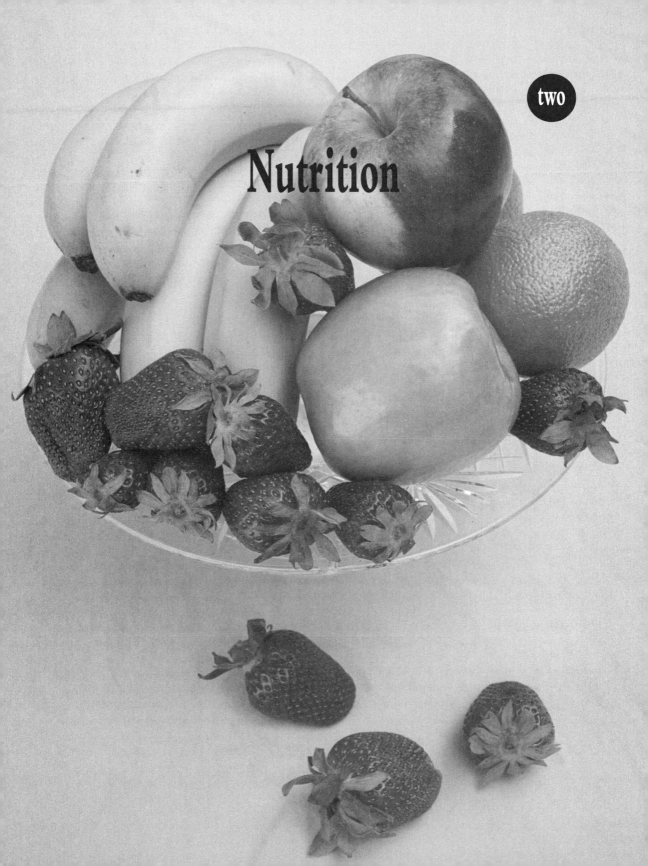

Nutrition

two

Eating for Optimum Health and Energy

In this chapter, Jackie Storm, Ph.D., C.N.S., provides her recommendations for a healthy nutritional plan that will leave you looking and feeling young:

Thirty years ago, the average women who walked into my office was twenty five years old and desperate to lose weight—by yesterday if possible. They often went so far as to say: "Just get the weight off me. I don't care if I'm healthy, I just want to be thin."

Today, the average woman who comes into my office is fifty five years old and having hot flashes. She still wants to be thin, but she also wants to be healthy. She's terrified of osteoporosis and swallowing enough calcium carbonate to turn her blood to cement. Her cholesterol is too high—according to her physician—who wants to put her on cholesterol-lowering medication, estrogen for the hot flashes and Fosamax for the osteoporosis.

As a clinical nutritionist and a behaviorist, my goal is to help my clients sort through the plethora of conflicting information, decide what to do, and make some appropriate changes. As a woman, I understand the issues on a personal as well as a professional level. I understand the pressure this society puts on us to be thin. I've also had the hot flashes, and I've wrestled with the health issues. I've seen the nutritional fads come and go, and I've seen the media messages that keep us in a total fog as to good and bad, right and wrong.

How sad it is that we measure our self-worth by the size of our thighs, rather than the condition of our hearts. I'm not referring to clogged arteries when I talk about the condition of our hearts. I'm thinking spiritually. Our hearts should be filled with love and compassion. Instead we stew in our anger, frustration and self-loathing.

So, where do I begin to tell you how to eat for optimum health and energy? What are the important nutrition principles we need to keep in mind, without getting bogged down in a lot of negativity?

- *First, let me suggest that you make an attempt to rediscover food.* Our Paleolithic ancestors were hunter-gatherers. They were nibblers rather than gorgers. They ate foods in season—real food—not refined flour and sugar products filled with hydrogenated fats, preservatives and chemicals. I am not suggesting that you give up every packaged food in existence forever and ever, but the foundation of your diet should consist of unprocessed foods.

- *Eat at regular intervals.* One of the biggest mistakes people make is to skip breakfast and go for long periods without food. When we first get up in the morning we are coming off of an overnight fast, and we need to put fuel in the tank. If we don't eat breakfast, metabolism has to slow down to compensate for the lack of fuel. When we finally get around to eating the body will over store what we consume, to get ready for the next famine. Rule of thumb: Don't go for more than five hours during the day without eating. If you aren't that hungry, eat lightly, but don't skip a meal.

- *Build your diet upon a foundation of protein.* Aim for three different high protein foods daily. Choices include: eggs, yogurt, cottage cheese, nuts, legumes, fish, chicken, lean meat, or tofu. Note: We are not aiming for quantity here. Side of cow? No way. A few ounces? Fine.

- *Learn to love fruits and vegetables.* Five a day, minimum. Nine a day would be even better if possible. Fruits and vegetables are your best source of vitamins, minerals, fiber, antioxidants and all the life-saving phytonutrients that keep making the news these days.

- *Go nuts. Have a handful of raw nuts*—cashews, walnuts, almonds —four to five times per week. Eat them as a snack, or add them to a salad. Nuts are an excellent source of essential fatty acids, as well as fiber, protein, and minerals like magnesium, potassium, and calcium. Peanuts, by the way, don't count here. They're legumes, not nuts.

- *Rediscover eggs.* Eggs are a neat little powerhouse of nutrition, in a portion-controlled package. They contain very good quality protein, plus choline, B vitamins, vitamin A and more. And eat the yolks. The cholesterol in your diet has virtually no impact on blood cholesterol, so enjoy.

- *Eat fish two or more times per week.* Fish is high in the essential fats (a.k.a. omega-3 fatty acids) that are so important for your heart and your immune system.

- *Eat off a salad plate.* If what you are having won't fit on a salad plate, it's probably too much food. One of the big problems with the American diet is that our portions have grown to gargantuan sizes. Switching to a salad plate is an easy way to control quantities without having to resort to counting calories.

- *Drink a glass of warm or room temperature water with a tablespoon of lemon juice before breakfast.* When we get up in the morning we are generally slightly dehydrated, so the water is an important ritual. The addition of lemon juice makes it a cleansing ritual. In addition, drink seven or more cups of liquid over the course of the day.

- *A yogurt a day keeps the doctor away.* This should be a natural yogurt with active yogurt cultures and no artificial sweeteners. The lactobacillus culture helps us to maintain the right kind of flora and fauna in our gut for optimum health and digestion. Alas, the over use of antibiotics leaves us vulnerable to an overgrowth of yeast and unhealthy bacteria that can lead to a variety of health problems, ranging from cystitis and vaginal yeast infections, to inflammatory conditions such as arthritis.

- *Take a high-potency multiple vitamin/mineral supplement to cover your BACES.* BACES is an acronym for B vitamins, plus vitamin A, C, E, and selenium. There is mounting evidence showing the benefits of supplementing with these important nutrients. Taking vitamins doesn't mean you can eat junk and not worry about it. The people who benefit most from supplements are those who already have a healthy diet.

- *Keep it simple.* In general, don't have more than three different foods at any one time. Forget the seven course meals.

- *Stop eating when you are no longer hungry, even if there is still food on the plate.*

Nutrition & Stress

One of the first recognizable symptoms of stress is often a change in eating habits. What the change consists of will vary from person to person, and from time to time. Some of us, when stressed, may find ourselves polishing off a bag of cookies. We are using food as a coping response. Others frequently find themselves relatively unable to eat when stressed. The variables here are (a) body type and (b) acute versus chronic stress.

Body Type

If you are physically high strung—which typically means thin, with low blood pressure—even modest amounts of stress will kill your appetite. Thin, high strung individuals have a lot of adrenaline flowing. Adrenaline is a stimulant, and stimulants are appetite suppressants. If your blood pressure tends to be low you will also be prone to adrenaline surges whenever your blood sugar drops.

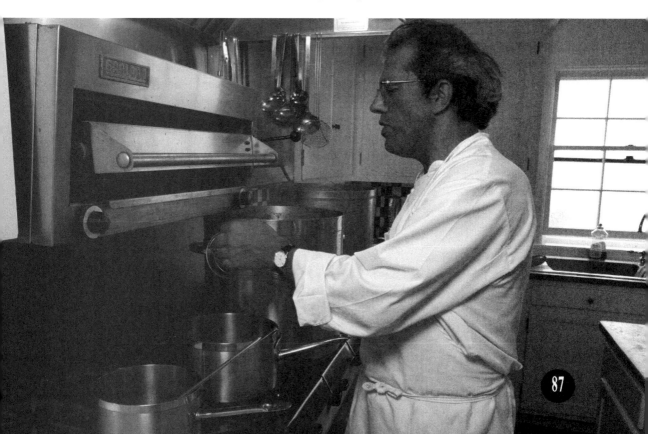

Live Long, Look Young!

If you have a stockier build you are more apt to use food as a coping response. Eating for you may activate the parasympathetic nervous system and bring on a relaxation response. Paradoxically, those who most need to eat, can't. (This is one of the reasons the thin stay thin.) Those who don't need food eat more and gain weight.

Acute vs. Chronic Stress

Chronic stress—the day-in, day-out petty annoyances and aggravations—is most apt to trigger an eating response. Acute stress—that's when the house burns down, you've just been fired from your job, and the dog is in the hospital—tends to take away the appetite of even the most dedicated chow hound. So much adrenaline is flowing during acute periods of stress that we can't eat. Typically people lose weight during times of acute stress.

Eating as a Coping Response

While it's true that eating helps to calm us, there are other reasons we reach for food when stressed:

- That's what we were taught to do as children. Think about it. The first time a baby cries in his crib someone sticks a bottle in his mouth. When we cry, we get a cookie, or a sweet. First trip to the dentist? Have a lollipop. First haircut? Have an ice cream cone.
- Food calms us physically. Food in the stomach diverts a certain amount of blood flow from the brain to the digestive tract. Hence, we get sleepy after a big meal. (This is why people pass out in their mashed potatoes after Thanksgiving dinner.)
- Food calms us biochemically. When we eat carbohydrates foods it tends to increase the brain's level of a neurotransmitter called serotonin. Serotonin has a calming, sleep-inducing effect. Some health professionals theorize that people who overeat carbohydrates—sugars and starches—are attempting to self-medicate. Unconsciously, they reach for carbohydrates in an effort to raise their serotonin level.

On a short term basis, if you have a few cookies at the end of a high stress day, it's no big deal. But on a long term basis, if you take in calories you don't need, you'll gain weight and/or develop health problems.

You can avoid eating to relieve stress by practicing other forms of relaxation. Treat yourself to a bubble bath, or a massage. Do some yoga stretches, and some breath meditation. Just because you learned to reach for food in response to stress, you're not stuck there. You can learn to do something else.

Let's look at some of the nutrients we may need more of because of stress:

VITAMIN C: Vitamin C is found in the body in two places: (1) our white blood cells, and (2) our adrenal glands. In the adrenal glands it helps in the production of stress hormones like epinephrine. Under high stress conditions it gets depleted. When that happens we are more susceptible to infection, and to bruising, bleeding, and even hemorrhage.

MAGNESIUM: Magnesium has many functions in the body—literally hundreds—including the production of energy, the manufacture of certain neurotransmitters—like serotonin—and regular heartbeat. It is magnesium that enables a muscle to relax after it has contracted. When we are stressed and the body releases epinephrine, our muscles often tense as part of the fight or flight response. When that happens, magnesium gets pulled out of our cells, and we can end up with a magnesium deficiency and muscles that are locked in tension. Many symptoms of stress—apathy, depression, forgetfulness, an inability to concentrate, muscle spasms, twitching, and a tendency to startle easily—are actually symptoms of magnesium deficiency.

Food sources of magnesium include chocolate and peanut butter. Magnesium is found in dark green vegetables, nuts and seeds, and legumes. Chocolate comes from the cocoa bean, and peanuts are goober peas, both members of the legume family.

PANTOTHENIC ACID: Vitamin B5 is needed for the production of epinephrine, which under high stress conditions gets depleted. So the more of it we have available the longer we will be able to produce epinephrine, and the longer we will last before we wear out, fall apart, get sick, or—God forbid—die.

ZINC: If the stress we are experiencing is physical—surgery, trauma, burn, or strenuous exercise—we will need more zinc. We need zinc to grow new skin cells, therefore we need it to heal.

Change Your Diet to Cope with Stress

Sometimes when we are stressed we feel wired, nervous and over stimulated. At other times, we feel fatigued, exhausted and unable to get out of bed. Certain body types are more apt to feel nervous and high strung, and certain other types are more apt to feel exhausted.

As a general rule, if you are feeling exhausted it is possible to increase your protein consumption in order to have more energy. Conversely, if you are high strung and you need to unwind, it is possible to increase your carbohydrate intake to raise your serotonin levels and calm yourself down. Please note that these are temporary changes to help you cope with the stress you are feeling at the moment. It is not intended that you follow an unbalanced regime on an ongoing basis.

Daily Food Guide for Healthy Adults

FRUITS: Two to three servings daily; choose fresh fruits in season.

VEGETABLES: Three servings daily. Make seasonal choices: raw, leafy greens in spring and summer; cooked root vegetables in fall and winter.

HIGH-PROTEIN FOODS: Choose three different foods daily from the following: Eggs, milk, yogurt, cottage cheese, fish, poultry, lean meat, nuts, seeds (or nut butters), tofu, legumes, protein shakes. Athletes and bodybuilders should increase to five servings daily.

GRAINS AND STARCHES: Choose whole grains and foods, such as oatmeal, sweet potato and legumes. Avoid refined processed starches made with white flower. Decrease consumption of starches to lose weight; increase to gain weight. Type II diabetics or people with Syndrome X (a cluster of symptoms including high blood pressure, glucose intolerance, high triglycerides and high cholesterol) may need to limit starch consumption to once a day.

FATS AND OILS: Include raw unsalted nuts and seeds in your diet. Olives and avocados are good choices. Choose olive oil or flaxseed oil for salad dressings. Use cold-pressed canola oil for cooking. Avoid hydrogenated fats, deep-fried foods, lard and processed meats.

Bernard Brulè—42 years young—Hamptons Private Chef

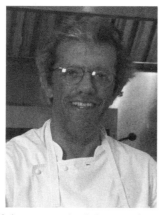

Bernard works as a private chef in Europe, Manhattan, and East Hampton, Long Island. He also teaches cooking classes to small groups of people in their homes. Bernard realizes that he benefits greatly from yoga class, it makes him feel less stressed, more peaceful and youthful. After his first class in a while, he felt achy. I told him to take another class soon, because with each class you feel better.

"I believe a person needs to find the right balance of exercise and do it regularly," says Bernard. Bernard likes to do yoga, meditate and fish in ponds, lakes and rivers. "Sometimes I eat what I catch, he explains. "But the main objective is releasing stress. No one is around and it is really a form of meditation. Just me and nature. When I feel an excess of energy, I like to go dancing."

In his cooking Bernard likes to use a moderate amount of spices so that they enhance, not overpower the flavors of the food. He likes to add his own French twist to different cuisines including Moroccan, Italian, Brazilian, and Indian. He also likes to travel to try different foods from around the world because it broadens his mind. Some cooking advice? "Try different flavors but don't mix too many ingredients and spices together. Simplicity is very important. Also, do not eat the same food all the time. In my cooking classes I recommend that people learn the basics, such as a stock that can be used in soup, sauces and recipes."

Bernard also has modified his approach. He used to use heavy cream and butter; now he uses low fat milk in a Vichyssoise, and sometimes substitutes olive oil for butter.

"I try to cook using local ingredients that are in season. Many of my clients request that I cook organically and always use the finest freshest ingredients."

Recipes

Here are a couple of great recipes that chef Bernard Brulè put together for you.

Grapefruit Granite (for six)

One quart of freshly squeezed pink grapefruit juice
One cup of granulated sugar
Juice of one orange

Mix the grapefruit juice with the sugar and the orange juice. Place it in a bowl in the freezer. Every hour or so mix the liquid with a fork until it becomes crystal.

Chicken Orientale (for six)

One chicken (approx. four pounds)

Flatten the chicken, cutting along the spine from the neck to the butt. Then squeeze four lemons, chop two white onions and five garlic cloves. Marinate the chicken for two hours by adding one cup of olive oil and one teaspoon of thyme. Roast the chicken in the oven at 475 degrees for forty five minutes. Add salt and pepper to taste.

Ratatouille

Chop six zucchini or yellow squash; peel one medium eggplant and soak in milk with pinch of salt.
Heat two tablespoons of olive oil in a saucepan. Sauté three cloves of minced garlic with one finely-chopped onion until onion is translucent. Add eggplant, zucchini, and one large can of chopped tomatoes. Simmer for one-half hour. Then, add one sprig of finely-chopped parsley and mint. Add salt and pepper to taste.

Lisa's Protein Shake

I make the following protein shake for my whole family: It's great in the morning or as a pick-me-up after a workout.

In a blender mix with ice: one scoop of protein powder, one cup of skim or soy milk, one banana or 1/2 cup of strawberries.

Juicing

Try one of the following combination juices after a workout.

High Energy Juice: carrot, beet, ginger and apple.
Liver Tonic: carrot, beet celery, grapefruit and apple.
Immune Builder: carrot, cucumber, beet and apple.

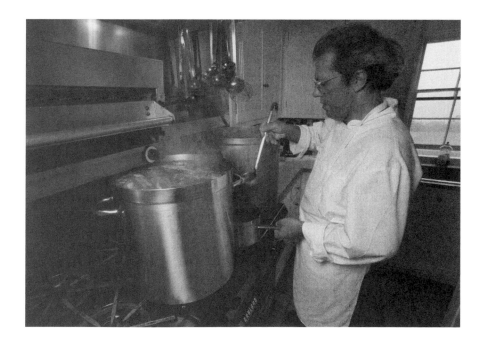

Enliven Your Senses with Tea

Tea drinking dates back 2500 years; today tea is the second most popular beverage in the world, with more than one-half billion cups of tea consumed each day! And for good reason. Drinking tea aids digestion, reduces headaches, enhances the immune system, reduces the risk of heart attack and stroke, and much more. Green teas are especially beneficial; they contain polyphenols that have proven health benefits. Asians are big tea drinkers and that habit is thought to be related to their longevity. Having a cup of tea with friends is rejuvenating and encourages the opening of consciousness. It energizes both the mind and spirit.

Recently, I met with Miriam Novelle, an entrepreneur who custom blends fragrances in teas. Miriam uses both her nose and knowledge to blend teas. She runs the best-known tea salon and emporium in the country. Located in New York City, it offers one of the largest selections of premium-blended teas in the world. When I met her for tea she had just finished packaging a tea for the Dalai Lama. She shared with me her knowledge of teas, explaining that teas are hand-picked from Camellia Sinuses then go through different processes that lead to varieties in teas.

GREEN TEAS: Yield a delicate flavor and aroma. They go through the lightest heating process. One of Miriam's strengths over the years has been introducing people to green teas, which have many nuances. She blends flowers, herbs and oils to create varieties and taste experiences.

OOLONG TEAS: Undergo a slightly longer oxidation period. The tea is a warm and golden color. A great Oolong tea has a soft peachy flavor.

BLACK TEAS: The leaves are allowed to fully oxidize. The liqueur results in a warm amber glow. There is a rich dry taste to the palette. Also, did you know that chamomile and mint tea are not really teas, but herbal infusions? They are drunk like teas but are in the herbal category.

Recently Miriam has introduced a meditation tea, which cultivates serenity. She recommends that we all take a few minutes out of our busy days to enjoy a cup of fine tea. Her philosophy about tea is evident in this poem:

There are times
When I've sat with a cup of tea
And drifted away.

There are times
When I've sat with a cup of tea
And contemplated the day.

There are times
When I've sat with a cup of tea
And wished for a longer day.

There are times
When I've just sat with a cup of tea.

—Miriam Novelle

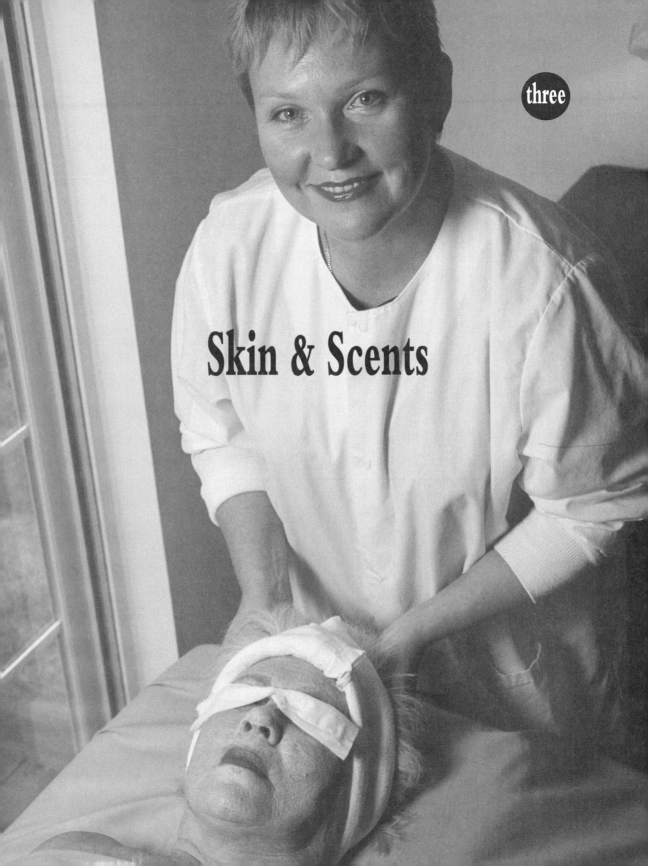

three

Skin & Scents

Skin Care

Nancy DePietro is a licensed esthetician with 20 years of experience, as well as a certified aromatherapist and healing touch practitioner, who runs her own practice in East Hampton, New York.

In this chapter, Nancy shares her knowledge on skin care and aromatherapy.

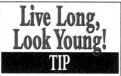

Loofa It

Loofa the skin of the legs, arms, torso and back before and after a shower. This exfoliates dry skin and enhances circulation.

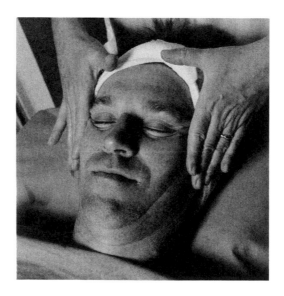

What's New In Skin Care

Let's start off talking about different skin types. All of us are born with a different genetic code that gives us our basic skin type: dry, sensitive, oily or combination. That said, the condition of our skin can change due to several factors. For example, in warmer humid climates our oil glands will tend to get activated and in colder dryer climates our skin may tend to get a bit dehydrated (water dry) and or slow down our oil glands. Illness and medications also affects the condition of skin as does smoking, excessive amounts of alcohol and unprotected sun exposure.

Since you know your skin better than anyone you need to ask yourself if you are doing all you can for it. Here are some tips: Make sure you are drinking plenty of healthful fluids, eating well, exercising, getting enough sleep, protecting your skin from the sun and not smoking.

Exposure to the sun's ultra violet (UV) rays is the major reason skin ages and increases your risk of skin cancer. Most people today are very aware of the danger and damage caused by unprotected and excessive sun exposure. Just take a look at your own skin. Look at the unexposed areas compared to those that are exposed. The exposed skin is discolored, less toned and wrinkled.

Sun damage is cumulative. The damage will show up as we age. It all starts with how well protected we were as children. Protect your children with a sunscreen year round with an SPF of 15 to 30. The UV is strongest between 10 a.m. and 4 p.m., so try to get out early in the morning or late in the afternoon. In addition to its effects on the skin, some scientists are concerned that UV exposure may impair the human immune system and increase the risk of cataracts and other eye problems.

This brings us right into the topic of wrinkles—although I call them character lines. The lines on a person's face and skin tone can tell us much about the physical and emotional health of an individual. We have determined that sun is the first major factor in breaking down the skin; age is the next. Starting at about age thirty, our oil glands start to slow down and we gradually lose our elasticity from a breakdown of collagen and elastin. We also lose a fat layer, which causes thinning of the skin.

We know how important nutrition is for our overall health. A healthful diet nourishes our skin, bringing nutrients to the blood stream. Nutritional needs vary depending on age, physical build and amount of daily exercise.

Sometimes in our busy lives we don't always eat sufficient quantities of the right foods and need to take supplements. Antioxidants play a very important role in the aging process both internally and topically. Topical products can provide higher concentrations of the vitamin to the skin. At one time the face and body creams on the market helped only the surface of the skin. In the last ten years breakthroughs in the cosmetic industry have brought it a new term called Cosmeceuticals. These are creams that penetrate to a deeper level to enhance the health and appearance of our skin.

Antioxidants

Vitamin E has been used in creams for years. It is a cellular antioxidant that protects skin from free radical damage. It is also very soothing and helps speed up the healing process. In the last decade researchers looked into other components of the vitamin—in particular Tocotrienols—and found them to be fifty times more powerful than other forms of vitamin E. Scientists then produced a liquid high in concentration of Tocotrienols, which are now being mixed into cosmetics.

I'm sure that by now most of you have been introduced to topical Vitamin C, a recent big breakthrough. Its main role is its antioxidant properties and it helps in the formation of collagen. It also has a toning and firming effect on the skin and can reverse a certain amount of damage caused by UVA and UVB rays, helping to diminish and soften fine lines. You will find two forms of Vitamin C on the market today; both are beneficial. One, L-ascorbic acid comes in serums or creams and different strengths: 10%, 15% and 20%. The other is Vitamin C Ester. This form is non-acidic and therefore non-irritating. It is recommended for very sensitive skin.

Vitamin A became popular in the 1970's. Available only by prescription, it was used as treatment for acne. Soon came the realization that it worked at a cellular level helping to increase collagen production. Retin-A is the new anti-aging cream. However, it may cause redness and increases sensitivity to sun exposure. More research brought about a less irritating formula called Renova with the same active ingredient as Retin-A in a less irritating base. Cosmetic companies then developed products with retinods that effectively improve the appearance of the skin without requiring a prescription. Vitamin A Palimate (a retinyl ester) is mostly used in the cosmetic industry. It is the least powerful, most stable and gets good results. All retinods are oil soluble and work synergistically with alpha hydroxy acid treatments, which are water-soluble. It is very effective to use one in the morning and one at night or to alternate daily.

Here is one antioxidant that may be less familiar but very important: alpha lipoic acid is an antioxidant that is both water and fat soluble. It fights free radicals in any part of a cell, and helps to protect Vitamin C and E. It also increases a cell's metabolism and capacity to heal, and is a very powerful anti-inflammatory. It is wonderful for sensitive skin.

DMAE (dimethylaminoethanol)—no wonder they abbreviated that one! Tough to say but a good one to remember. This is an antioxidant stabilizer that actually becomes part of the cell membrane, helping it to resist stress, and increasing circulation and tone.

Coenzyme Q10 (Co-Q10) has recently been used in topical skin creams for the treatment of aging skin. Co-Q10 is found in all cells of our body and assists in cellular metabolism and energy production. It is a powerful, fat-soluble antioxidant that protects our skin from free radical damage and oxidative stress.

This is one that I'm sure most of you are familiar with—alpha hydroxy acids (AHA) In the 1990's they became very popular in the medical and skin care fields. Unknowingly however, people have been benefiting from it for ages: French and Italian women used to wash their faces with aged wine and the Egyptians took baths in sour milk to condition their skin. AHA's are derived from citrus fruits, green tea, apples and fruit acid products. These acids are mild and help to increase cell renewal. Green tea extract acts as an anti-irritant and works well when combined with fruit acid concentrations.

AHA's weaken the bonds that hold dead skin together resulting in an exfoliation of dead skin cells and quicker growth of new skin cells. It leaves your skin smoother and rejuvenated. Research and clinical studies are finding that long-term use of AHA's may also increase collagen production.

Aromatherapy

After studying aromatherapy in 1985 I incorporated it into my skin care practice with therapeutic results. It has become a way of life for me. Aromatherapy is a holistic approach for healing the body, mind and spirit. It is based on the awareness that high-grade essential oils help to create emotional, physical and energetic balance.

The essences are extracted from wild and organic plants, which have great therapeutic value and are the most active and balanced. Aromatherapy helps us in many ways. Not only does it treat the condition of your skin, it also treats stress symptoms, anxiety, sleep disorders, muscle pain, etc. Through inhalation, the vapors are absorbed by the olfactory nerves affecting the limbic system, which connects the hypothalamus, pituitary glands, adrenal glands and sexual glands. The vapors also stimulate your memory center, affect your emotions, your appetite and much more. When you inhale the vapors through your mouth, their essence is absorbed through blood vessels in the lungs, affecting the entire respiratory system. Applied directly to the skin they are easily absorbed within ten minutes, penetrating the muscles, joints and organs.

When using essential oils, precautions need to be taken. Therapeutic grades of essences are very powerful and you should always seek out a qualified aromatherapist for guidance. Certain oils should never be used on pregnant women, while breast feeding or on infants and young children. Also, take caution if you suffer from asthma or certain allergies. Know your supplier. You will only get therapeutic results from high-grade organic essential oils.

All essential oils need to be diluted in vegetable oil to be effective and safe before being applied to the skin. Use one to two drops less than one teaspoon of vegetable oil for face oil; 5-10 drops per tablespoon of body oil and ten to twenty drops for bath oil.

Essential Oils for Aromatherapy

Especially good to live long and look young. Recommended by aromatherapist Robin Schierenbeck of Mood Beauty in East Hampton.

BASIL: clearing and strengthening, excellent nerve tonic, clears mind, aids in concentration.

BERGAMOT: uplifting and refreshing, good for depression and nervous tension, useful in skin care.

BLACK PEPPER: useful as a muscle rub after exercise.

CHAMOMILE FRANCE: soothing, gentle, relaxing oil, excellent for many skin conditions, soothes burns, inflamed wounds, calms hypersensitive skin and super allergic conditions.

CLARY SAGE: ultra-relaxing, used for muscle and nervous tension.

CYPRESS: toning and astringent, good for foot baths.

EUCALYPTUS: clearing and antiviral, used for colds and flus.

FRANKINCENSE: rejuvenating, good for mature skin, deeply relaxing, used for meditation.

GERANIUM: balancing, regulating, good for balancing female hormones, used in skin care.

GINGER: warming and fortifying muscle tonic, aids digestion, good for aches and pains.

GRAPEFRUIT: uplifting and refreshing, good for stress, great in baths, a good pick-menu.

JASMINE EGYPT: luxurious, relaxing, sensuous, calming, lifts mood, boosts self-esteem, highly effective tonic for dry, sensitive skin. Alluring scent, smells different on everyone; great on men.

JUNIPER BERRY: diuretic, cleansing and detoxifying, used for cellulite treatments.

LAVENDER BULGARIAN: relaxing and healing, excellent for headaches, stress, burns, insect bites, insomnia, tension, anti-inflammatory, super soothing during mood changes (One to two drops can be applied directly to an area.)

LEMON: antiseptic and astringent, great hair rinse.

LIME: activating and stimulating, good for apathy, anxiety and depression, uplifts tired minds.

MELISSA: calming and regulating, pleasant to burn in the house.

NEROLI TUNISIAN: calming and soothing, ideal for skin care, especially mature, dry skin, helps restore sleep, relieves chronic states of anxiety, instills sense of peace.

ORANGE: soothing, warming great for the winter months.

PALMAROSA: uplifting, calming, clarifying, helpful for stress and tension.

PATCHOULI: relaxing and sensual, exotic and musty, excellent for healing all types of skin.

ROSE MOROCCO: healing, used for anger, grief, bereavement, and empathetic to all emotions, mental exhaustion, mild depression, grief, jealousy, resentment, nervous tension. On skin soothes mature, dry, sensitive or damaged skin, softens everything (including the heart!)

ROSEMARY: stimulating, relieves muscular fatigue, clears the mind.

SANDALWOOD: sedative, comforting, useful in meditation.

TANGERINE: soothing, good for the digestive and nervous system.

VETIVERT: calming, sedative and soothing, good for stress tension and joint mobility.

Live Long, Look Young!

YLANG YLANG: sensual sweet and exotic, used as an aphrodisiac, and as a softening skin care product.

SPECIAL MOOD-BEAUTY-FACE-OIL: blends apricot, camellia, wheat germ, jojoba, grape seed base oil with lavender and chamomile essential oils.

Recommendations For Using Special Oils

- Do not use undiluted on skin
- Do not take internally
- Keep out of reach of children and pets
- Keep away from eyes
- If pregnant or epileptic, seek medical advice
- Store in a cool, dark place
- Keep cap lightly closed

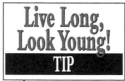

Sniff This

Put a couple of drops of essential oil on a handkerchief and breathe in deeply. Oil of basil is said to increase memory, while peppermint energizes and lavender relaxes.

Facials

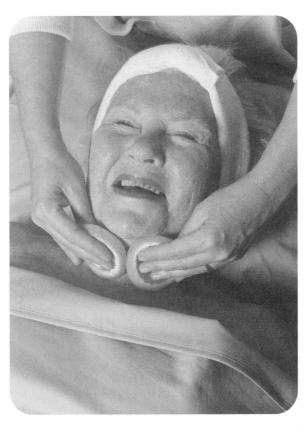

Looking back, I am so thrilled at how the skin industry has grown. When I first started out as a licensed hairdresser and decided to study to become a licensed esthetician, facials were not as popular as they are today. Although they were a norm in Europe, in the United States only big cities with top salons and spas offered facial treatments. Today it's hard to find a salon that doesn't offer a variety of facials.

Facials today are much more than a luxury. They are relaxing and benefit the client physically as well as psychologically. They help to maintain the health of the skin and correct any skin conditions, increase the circulation of the blood to nourish the skin, increase cell metabolism, activate the glands in the skin, and help to soften and prevent the formation of wrinkles and other signs of aging.

One common question is how often should one receive a facial. That all depends on your skin. Normal healthy skin will benefit from a facial every four to six weeks. If that is difficult to do, I strongly suggest at least four times a year seasonally. Problem skin will get positive results from facials given every week to every other week. Once the problem is corrected a monthly facial is recommended. Aging skin benefits from monthly treatments to condition and improve the texture of the skin. If your facial includes peeling treatments, a series of six to ten will provide the best results.

Live Long, Look Young!

The European Facial

This facial is designed to restore balance to the skin, to exfoliate and to deeply cleanse the pores. The esthetician will first determine the needs of your skin. Then she will use products to target your individual needs. There will be steam involved, and a facial massage. There may or may not be other facial equipment used, such as a light vacuum to help loosen embedded impurities in the pores. This is followed with manual extraction to remove gently any whiteheads or blackheads. After that a penetrating mask is applied. Sometimes during the mask your hands and feet are massaged and you are given heated mittens and booties to wear. After removal of the mask, the proper skin care products are applied and you leave feeling relaxed, clean and with the softest skin ever.

Aromatherapy Facial

This is sixty to ninety minutes of total relaxation, and is the most holistic approach to using natural ingredients as the essential oils quickly absorb into the skin and are very powerful. It uses high grade organic essential oils to support the skin's functions on a cellular level, helping to nourish, stimulate, detoxify and balance the skin. By inhaling the vapors of the essences it also becomes therapeutic on an emotional level. You will see and feel the results immediately. Your esthetician/aromatherapist will determine which essences to use to help to restore balance to your skin and will also give you steam and a massage concentrating on the lymph system. Deep pore cleansing and a mask with essential oils are added. Hands and feet are massaged while the mask is on, also concentrating on the lymph system to aid in tissue detoxification.

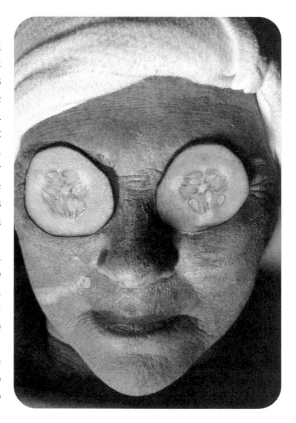

Lymph Drainage Facial

This facial aids circulation and detoxifies tissues. It helps reduce fluid retention and puffiness and stimulates the immune system. It is rejuvenating to the skin and helps to soften the appearance of fine lines and deeper wrinkles. The lymph system is the drainage system for the body's tissues. The lymph is a clear watery fluid that circulates through the lymphatic system carrying nourishment from the blood to the cells and removing waste from the cells. This system parallels the blood circulation but doesn't have the help of the heart pump. It depends on movement and pressure from the activity of the muscles. A complete lymph drainage massage in a facial treatment starts with the chest and neck area, working its way up. It takes approximately twenty to thirty five minutes.

The Oxygen Facial

This treatment is very helpful for dehydrated, sluggish, acne and hyperpigmented skin. Steam is applied and massaged with an oxygenated cream with vitamins, minerals and essences. This is followed by a light exfoliation. Oxygen is than passed over the skin providing rehydration and balancing.

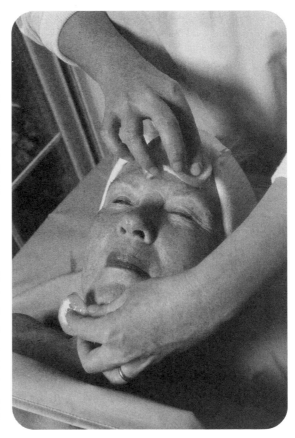

Enzyme Peels

With their synergistic blend of fruit enzymes, such as papaya and pineapple to loosen skin debris, these facials benefit all skin types. They remove dead skin cells speeding up cell renewal, restore tone, smooth skin structure, and help to lighten hyperpigmentation. An enzyme peel leaves your skin feeling smoother and radiant.

AHA Peeling Treatments

These non-aggressive, exfoliating treatments gently ease away fine lines and uneven texture and hyperpigmentation. AHA's fruit acids and glycolic acids weaken the bonds that hold dead skin cells together resulting in visible cell renewal and rejuvenation. They also help to dissolve debris from clogged pores.

Microdermabrasion

This is the latest treatment available. It exfoliates a little deeper than the above treatments. It is a painless procedure with no down time and uses an air-powered flow of aluminum crystals. To get the best results a weekly series of six to ten treatments should be done. Having this procedure just twice a year will dramatically slow down the aging process!

What About Men?

Can men benefit from facial treatments and all the lotions and potions on the market today? You bet! It is true that men's skin is different from women's skin. Men have thicker skin and their oil glands produce more oil. As we age, both men and women experience hormonal changes. Women lose estrogen and men lose testosterone, leaving both with thinner skin. Women just lose it faster and have more delicate skin. Men need to use precaution when exposed to sun and other extreme weather conditions. They also are affected by free radical damage, stress, nutritional needs, sleep and regular exercise. Men's thicker skin and larger pores get congested and benefit from a deep pore-cleansing facial. In addition, shaving tends to cause breakouts, ingrown hairs and razor burn. A soothing facial treatment with some guidance on skin care needs would do wonders. The next time you are in search of a gift for that special guy in your love life treat him to a facial or, better yet, a day at a spa!

four

Massage

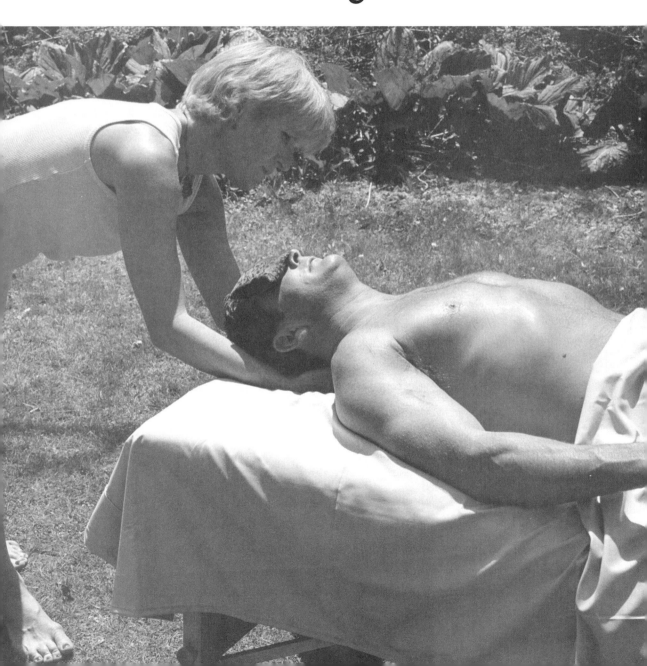

The Benefits of Massage

Massage is a relaxing, loving, and healing treatment. Like yoga, massage helps us to make the connection between the mind, body and spirit. Pain is usually caused by lack of oxygen and circulation, and can disappear when oxygen is restored. Massage releases toxins that are trapped in clogged lymph passages and increases the flow of oxygen throughout the body. After an exercise session, massage helps to release the build up of lactic acid in the muscles that also can lead to pain and discomfort. It helps bring your body to its most healthful and youthful state. Massage is extremely relaxing and rejuvenating for the body, mind and spirit.

It is important to take time out for yourself. In this book I specifically address self- massage. There are many other types of massage. Nothing can replace the benefits of scheduling a full body massage.

As we talk about in the section on yoga, there are overlapping benefits of massage and yoga. First, they both help to relieve tension and stress. Sometimes you are mentally or emotionally tired and fatigued, and your muscles ache. At these times you can benefit from the healing hands of a well trained Massage Therapist. At other times you might have over exerted yourself or pulled a muscle and massage can release the knots, sending more circulation to the blocked areas.

When you receive a massage, you let go of worries as the physical knots are released. You tune into the deep breathing techniques that are taught in yoga. Sometimes, the practitioner will play relaxing music and use aromatherapy. All this puts us into a meditative healing state. The feeling you have after a massage is very similar to how you feel after a yoga class.

I am a Licensed Massage Therapist as well as a Certified Yoga Instructor. When I teach a yoga class I often incorporate some self-massage techniques like working on your feet when you are in the butterfly posture, or doing some facial massage in the lotus (cross-legged) position. During massage treatments I encourage my clients to take full, deep breaths to enhance relaxation and to tune into the areas we're working on. This helps release tension and enhances awareness so that they can feel the positive changes in their bodies. In addition, I stretch my clients on the table and teach them yoga poses that they can add to their workouts.

Massage Styles

To experience the art of massage, you can make an appointment with a Licensed Massage Therapist. Everyone should do this: whether four times a year, once a month or every week. You can select a therapist that specializes in a particular style of massage, or one that combines several techniques. In my practice I combine Swedish, Trigger Point, Reflexology and Aromatherapy. Recently, I have been going to a Massage Therapist who combines Stone and Swedish massages. When you find a Massage Therapist that you like, you should continue with him or her. Over time, you build up trust and the therapist learns what works best for you.

Here is a description of some of the techniques used by the different types of massages. They all provide a sense of relaxation, healing and well being, as well as eliminate and reverse the effects of stress.

SWEDISH: Long strokes, kneading, friction and tapotement are combined to increase circulation and to aid the lymphatic system.

SHIATSU: A system of applying pressure with the thumb or elbow along the meridians.

MEDICAL: Concentrated friction and lymphatic drainage to promote healing.

CRANIAL SACRAL: Techniques done primarily on the head and pelvis to balance the flow of spinal fluid.

REFLEXOLOGY: Techniques done on the hands and the feet to enhance relaxation and balance energy throughout the body.

HOT STONE: Long strokes using stones that are hot enough to warm and relax the body. Stones are placed on lymphatic points to increase circulation. Sometimes, they are placed on chakras (energy centers) to enhance relaxation and meditation.

REIKI: An energy healing modality that involves chanting and hands-on healing. Lucia provides more on this wonderful practice.

Live Long, Look Young!

In addition to getting a professional massage, you can exchange massages with a friend. It can be a wonderful way to communicate. I often invite a friend over and we exchange massage. (Of course, I am lucky to have friends who know a lot about massage). Anyone can learn the basic techniques to give a friend or family member a wonderful, relaxing massage. The following photos show the basic Swedish Massage strokes:

Swedish Massage

Exchange with a friend. Find a quiet serene place. Work on a yoga mat at a massage table. Apply oil or lotion to your hands and rub it onto the entire back.

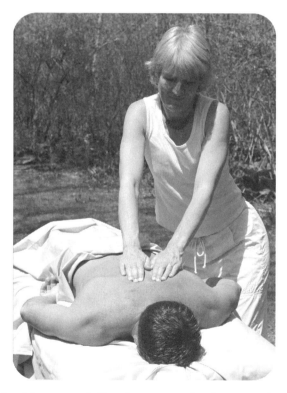

EFFLEURAGE A: Use your full palms to make long strokes up the back and around the shoulders. Then lightly stoke down the back three times.

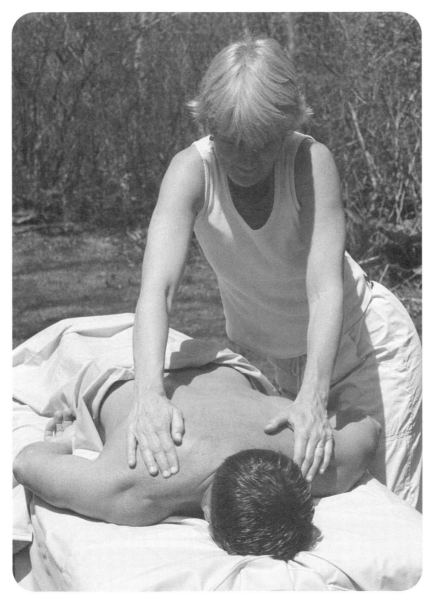

EFFLEURAGE B: Begins to warm up the muscles. It is a good stroke to repeat throughout the massage.

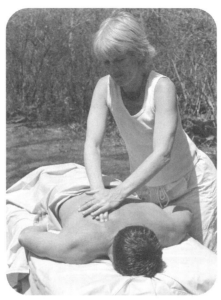

PETRISSAGE: This kneading movement involves making circles with the palms on the spine. The stroke roles and squeezes the muscles increasing circulation.

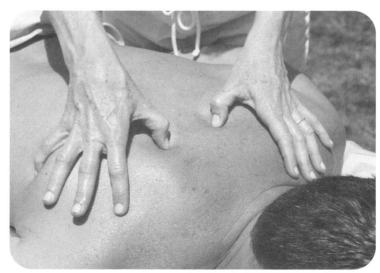

KNEADING: Concentrate on tight areas, making small circles there until the muscles loosen a bit.

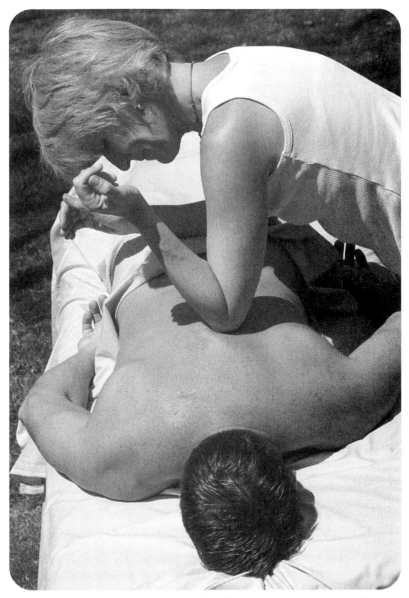

ELBOW EFFLEURAGE: Along the side of the spine, use your elbow to glide up and down the muscle. Be sensitive to how much pressure you apply. Get feedback from your partners.

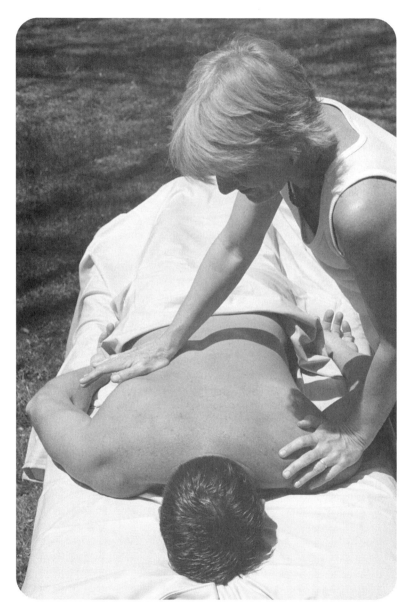

TRANSVERSE STRETCH: Place on hand on one hip the other on the opposite shoulder. Stretch on the exhale.

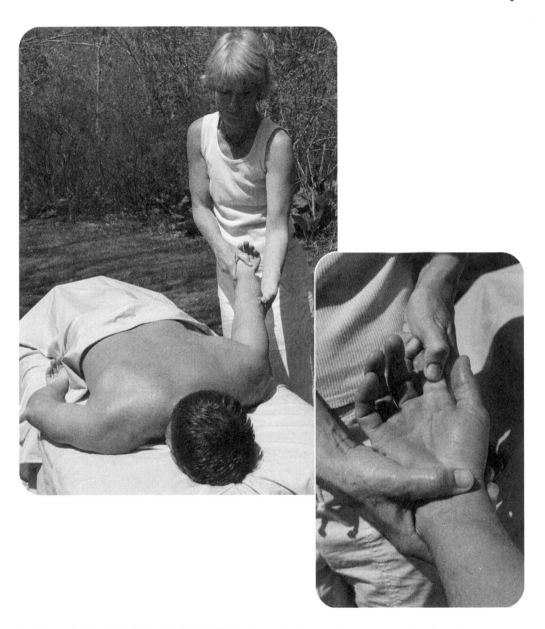

ARM AND FINGER STRETCH: Stretch down the arms to the hand. Massage the palm with small circular strokes. Pull and lengthen each finger.

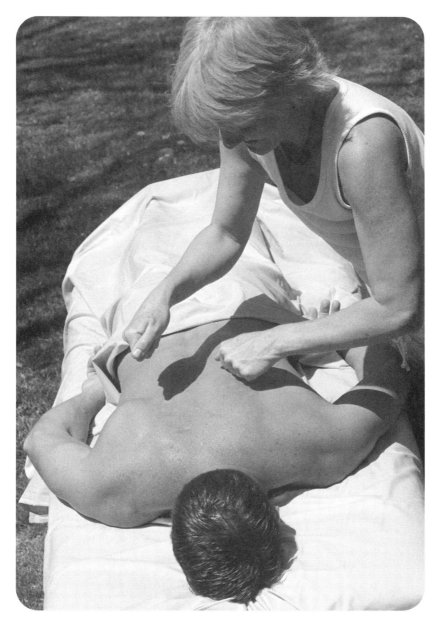

TAPOTEMENT: Simulate playing the drums with fingertips or fists. Lightly tapping the entire back in order to stimulate the muscle.

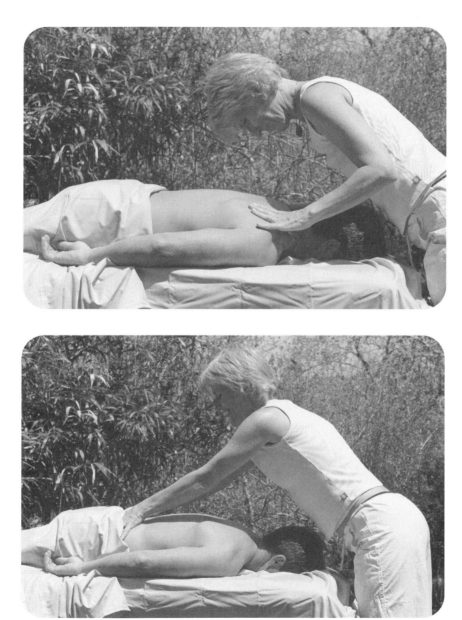

EFFELURAGE: Long stroke with full palms from the top of the shoulder down to the hips and back three times.

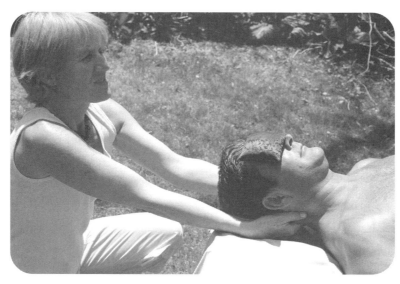

NECK STRETCH: Hook your fingertips under the ridge of your partner's head. Hold while you support his neck and tilt his head.

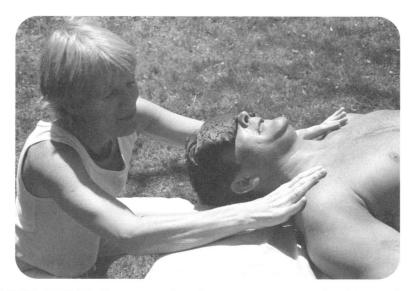

SHOULDER PRESS: Bring your hands to your partner's shoulder and press into the shoulders with your thumbs. Sense where there might be tension and press in that area three to five times.

Massage can be practiced between friends and lovers. It is a wonderful, sensual art. People learn to give and to receive pleasure. It feels great and has so many health benefits!

Benefits of Massage

- Relieves mental and physical stress
- Aids the lymphatic system
- Expands range of motion
- Enhances mental clarity and alertness
- Improves attention span
- Increases circulation and vitality
- Slows down aging/rejuvenates the body
- Prevents injuries
- Relieves muscle strain
- Increases flexibility
- Reduces fatigue
- Balances the nervous system
- Increases energy and endurance
- Balances emotions
- Nurtures the spirit

Self-Massage

Learn these basic techniques of self-massage to relieve tension. If you feel a headache coming on or if your eyes are tired, try the facial self-massage. The foot massage is great if your feet are tired or if your back is tight.

I also encourage you to try some self massage during yoga. For example, while in the butterfly pose you can do some reflexology by massaging the arches of your feet. Notice where you feel sensitive and make small circles there with your thumbs. At the end of a yoga class, or when at home practicing guided relaxation, you can use your fingertips to lightly massage your temples and eyebrows. You'll feel great!

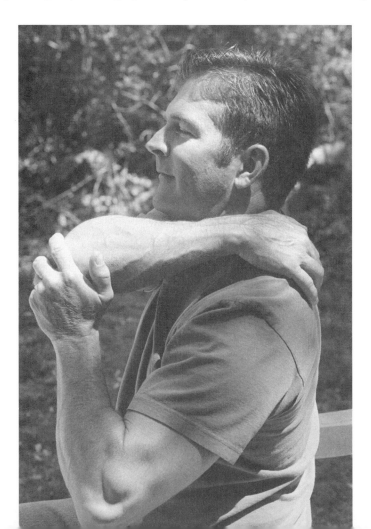

Facial Self-Massage

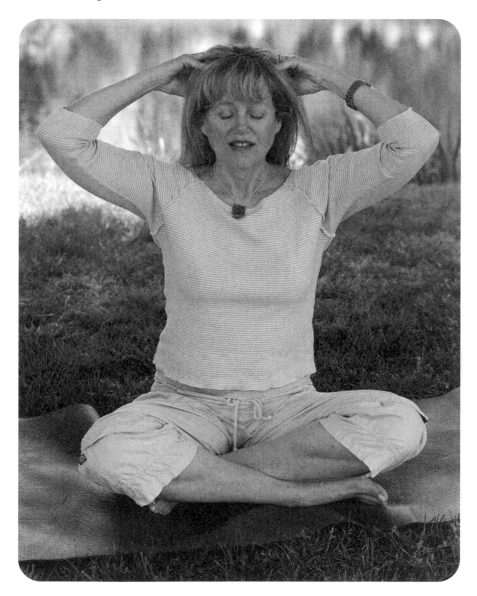

SCALP: Make small circles with your fingertips on your scalp and massage your head as if you are doing a deep shampoo.

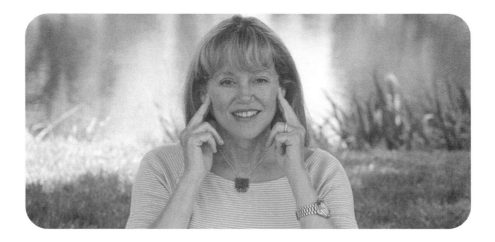

JAWS: Use your two index fingers and palce them on your jaw joint to make small circles. Three in one direction and three in the other direction.

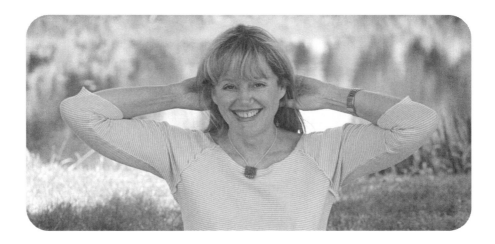

NECK RELEASE: Use your finger tips to make small circles where the neck and head meet.

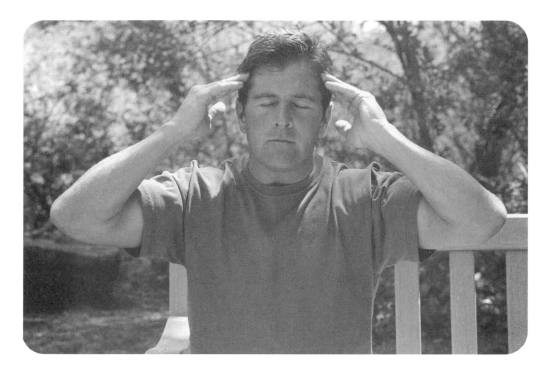

TEMPLES: Place your index and middle fingers on your temples and lightly masage up and down. (This is great for relieving headaches).

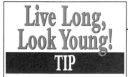

Ease Your Ears

With your fingertips, massage in gentle circles around your temples and ears. The ears are a microcosm of the entire body. There are over one hundred reflexology points located in your ears that are connected to and help energize different organs and parts of the body.

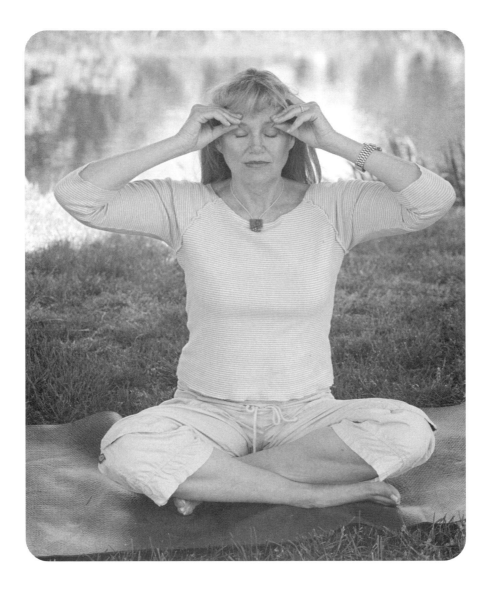

EYEBROW SQUEEZE: Squeeze your eyebrow between your thumb and index fingers, moving from the inner brow to the outer.

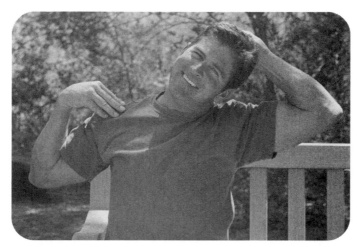

NECK AND SHOULDER STRETCH: Tilt head to the right place. Right hand above the left ear. Left hand on the left shoulder. Breathe and gently stretch. Repeat on the other side.

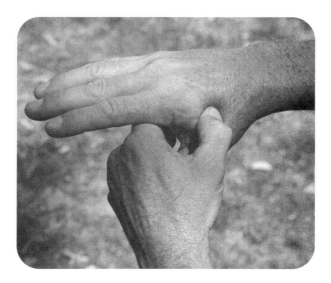

HAND POINT: Use the thumb and index finger of one hand to massage the web of your other hand (the space in between your thumb and index finger.) This massage is particularly helpful for people who suffer from repetitive stress syndrome such as carpal tunnel.

Reflexology

Reflexology is centuries old. Techniques were practiced thousands of years ago in Japan, India, Russia and Egypt. For years, feet have been worked on to promote wellness. These techniques are now used by practitioners in the modern day practice of reflexology. Reflexology is a form of massage that reduces stress and improves physical well-being and is based on the concept that parts of your body correspond to vital organs and nerves.

For example, there are reflexes on your feet that correspond to all the major organs, glands and body parts. The bottom of your foot contains a map of the entire body; there are 7000 nerve endings called reflexes, each of which corresponds to an organ or nerve in your body. Simply pressing a point on your foot can cause a response that helps to soothe, balance and relax your entire body.

Reflexology increases circulation and gently balances the nervous system. It clears the energy pathways that run throughout the body. A weakness or imbalance somewhere in

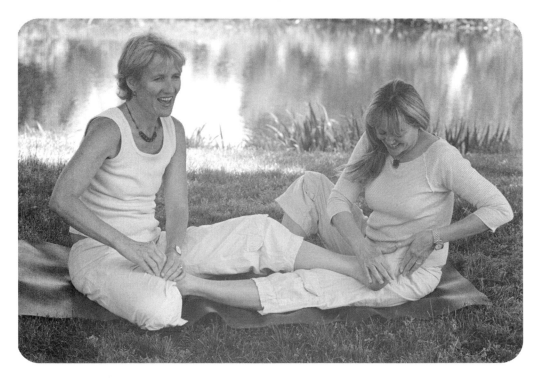

the body may be experienced as tenderness in the corresponding area of the foot. I know from the experience of working on many feet that reflexology works. Also, reflexology relaxes the mind and this is so basic to relaxation.

Once you can relax your mind, the body follows. If you feel overtired, reflexology works wonders to rejuvenate you. In addition, reflexology is very effective for overcoming jet lag. It induces such a deep state of relaxation that you may feel like you have just awaken from a refreshing long nap!

Reflexology is so relaxing and easy for a beginner to learn. Simply by starting to massage your friend's feet you start to relax them—as long as you work deeply enough and don't tickle them! If your friend laughs, which in itself is very healing, ask him or her to take deep full breaths, and then massage a little deeper. When my clients have ticklish or extremely sensitive feet, I encourage them to take long yoga breaths and they slowly relax and enjoy the effects of reflexology. There are many wonderful creams you can use during the massage. Some lotions are made specifically for foot massage. I like to use peppermint foot cream which leaves a cool refreshed feeling on the feet.

I recommend that you first receive a professional reflexology treatment to experience the deep effects of a complete treatment. Then, try the simple techniques I present below on a friend.

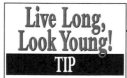

Share Touch

Sit with a friend on the couch or on the floor and exchange foot massage. Follow directions on page and then improvise.

Basic Techniques of Reflexology

Have the person you are working on lie down or sink back into a comfortable position.

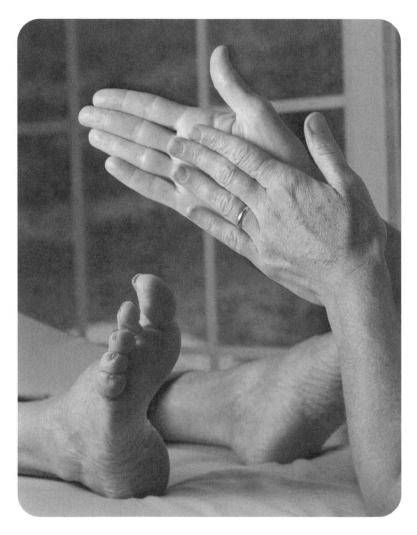

1. **WARM UP HANDS:** Warm up some lotion in your hands. Put lotion on the entire foot. Start at the ankle and rub out through the toes.

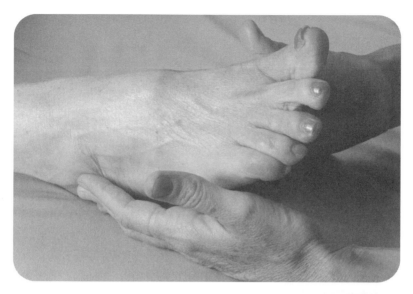

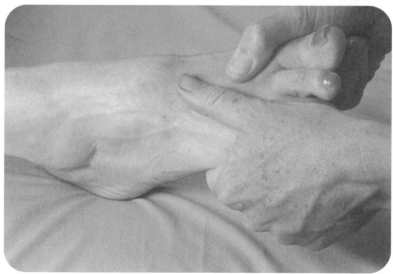

2. CIRCLE ANKLES AND STROKE UP FOOT: Place your thumbs on the heel and ankles and make small circles. Press your thumbs into different reflexes for a few seconds then make small circles. If a point seems particularly sensitive, it may need a little more work to release congestion. Stroke up the foot.

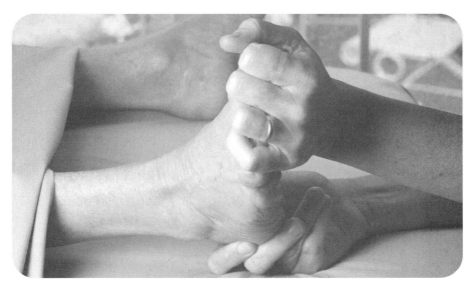

3. **ROTATE ANKLES:** Support the foot. One hand on the toes, one hand on the ankle. Rotate three times to the left, then three times to the right.

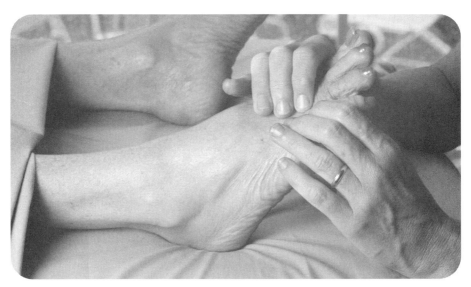

4. **MASSAGE IN BETWEEN TOES:** Massage in between the bones at the top of the foot with fingertips.

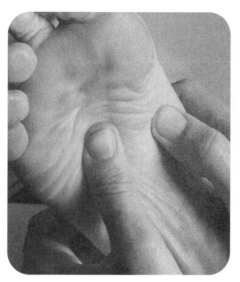

5. **THUMB CIRCLES ON BOTTOM:** Place your thumbs on the bottom of the foot and make small circular movements. Especially making circles along the arch of the foot.

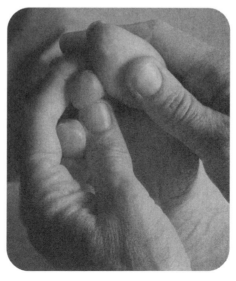

6. **MASSAGE TOES:** With a kneading motion, massage out through each toe.

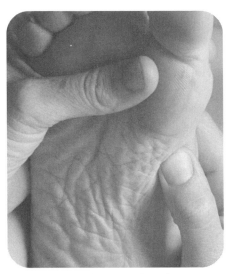

7. **THUMB PRESS UP ARCH:** With your thumb press up through the arch. The arch corresponds to the spine.

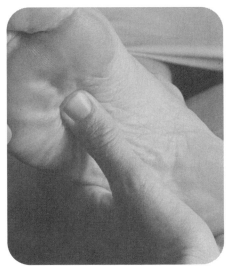

8. **SOLAR PLEXUS POINT:** Press against the Solar Plexus Point (at the center of the bottom of both foot, right beneath your toes). This helps to relax the diaphragm muscle, enabling more complete breathing. This massage can be done at the beginning and at the end of a reflexology session.

Benefits of Reflexology

- Revitalizes body
- Cleanses the body of toxins and impurities
- Enhances wellness
- Nurtures relationships

- Relaxes the mind
- Releases muscles in the back
- Increases circulation throughout the body
- Relieves emotional stress

Facial Rejuvenation

Facial rejuvenation treatments, in which fragrant wraps are pressed into your skin, ease and help to erase the signs of aging and stress. Beauty does come from within, but it is important to feel relaxed. We all need to work on ourselves internally but pampering and setting time aside for someone to help you rejuvenate is also important.

Facial rejuvenation connects to the emotional self. It helps you to release the energy that holds feelings that no longer serve you. The belief is that feelings take the physical form of emotional crystallizations in your cells. This tension is held and is visible in your face through muscular contractions that hold traumas from your past. During facial rejuvenation, the whole body experiences a deep state of relaxation and the contractions are released.

Facial rejuvenation is a form of reflexology so that during the facial rejuvenation treatment, you are working your twelve major nerve centers. Your face, head and entire body receive healing benefits. Facial rejuvenation combines massage strokes and trigger points, using healing organic oil blends. A masque is applied to draw out toxins and tone your facial muscles. Your face looks relaxed, refreshed and radiant after a treatment and the benefits last long afterwards. Your face, neck and shoulders gain tone and flexibility. The skin cells are nourished with increased flow of oxygen, blood and lymph. Nerve pathways open throughout the head, neck and body, enhancing a free flow of circulation. Facial rejuvenation firms and realigns your facial muscles. As emotional crystallizations held in your musculature dissolve, you regain full responsiveness and expression in the face. You regain your youthful expression and tone.

Live Long, Look Young! PROFILE — Lucia Hwong—Reiki Master

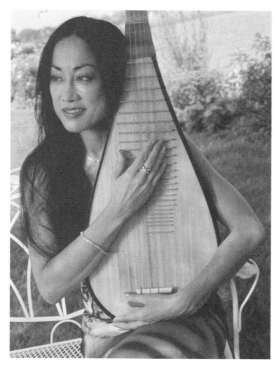

Lucia shares her secrets to staying young and living to your fullest potential.

Finding the joy in every moment, movement and thought. Love always puts a glow in your cheeks. Don't wait for love to find you; create it wherever you are. Surround yourself with people whom you love and create a mutually supportive network. Do something that becomes a bright light in someone's life and gives them joy; it can be as easy as a smile.

Do something for yourself that gives you joy in your soul. Take a moment to enjoy the colors of a sunrise or sunset.

Take a deep breath and let it fill you with energy and fulfillment. Surround yourself with beauty by seeing beauty in everything.

Make the most of the gifts you already have in your life. As you give thanks for all the positive aspects of your life, it brings more abundance. Be creative and acknowledge even the smallest detail that makes you special.

Whatever you choose to do, from practicing yoga, to starting a business, it is all about discovery and revelation. "I try to cook using local ingredients that are in season. Many of my clients request that I cook organically and always use the finest freshest ingredients."

An Interview with Lucia Hwong

What is Reiki?

Reiki is a spiritual and healing modality that tunes you into universal unconditional love. The healing and transformational energy of this universal love is transmitted through chants, hands-on healing and symbols. The practice of Reiki increases the balance of the life-force that resides in all of us so that the body, mind and spirit can function harmoniously. It is a conscious practice of creating a loving and nurturing environment at every moment—especially when things are difficult. I came to study Reiki when my father was ill with cancer. He had meditated most of his life and used meditation to regain strength after chemotherapy treatments. After meditating for a few days, he would be strong enough to travel with my mother and they would schedule their return home to his next chemotherapy treatment. During the last few months of his life he was too weak to sit up and meditate.

I knew that meditating was so important to calm and center him that I decided to study a practice in which I could channel life force energy for him. Friends introduced me to Reiki, which in Japanese and Chinese means "universal life energy" or "supernatural energy." It is a powerful form of hands-on healing discovered 100 years ago by Dr. Mikao Usui, who was researching the healing and transformational methods used by history's greatest healers, including Jesus Christ and Buddha. He discovered the Tibetan Lotus Sutras which included both vocal mantras and hand mudras for healing. He passed his knowledge on to his students Chujiro Hayashi and Hawayo Takata, the latter of whom brought Reiki to America.

Reiki has been developed into a powerful tool that includes the use of sound and visual symbols to increase the balance and life force that resides in all living things so that the body, mind and spirit function harmoniously. It is not a religious; it is a spiritual practice that stimulates one's own natural healing powers. Anyone can learn how to perform Reiki by attending a Reiki school, two of which are mentioned in the resources section of this book.

When I gave him Reiki sessions I could see how this universal life energy traveled through me, lifted his spirit and gave him tranquility. Part of the beauty of Reiki also is that when I gave the sessions, the universal life energy traveling through me opened my

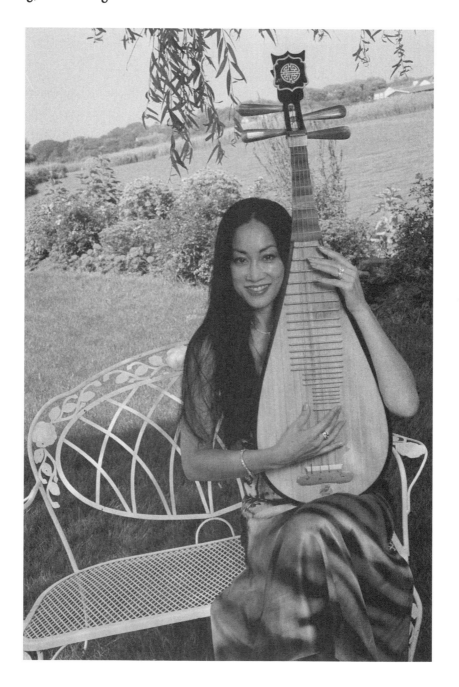

heart with love. Whenever people around me are in distress I send them Reiki energy for balance, love and empowerment.

Explain how you incorporate music into Reiki?

After my father passed away, I wanted to share the power of Reiki healing energy through an art form I have studied since I was a child—music. I composed the Goddess CDs with music which has Reiki chants woven into it. My intention is for the music to provide the listener with virtual Reiki sessions for well being. The rhythms and melodic patterns are based on the pulses and tones that I hear when I am in the meditative Reiki state of unconditional love.

Through my father's illness I discovered the healing energy of Reiki and incorporated it into my music and life. That is the amazing journey of life; a profoundly sad event can become a pivotal point of transformation.

How do you recommend dealing with life's challenges?

If something negative happens around you, find the energy to turn it into a positive. If someone expresses anger see if there is a way to resolve the root of their anger. If I feel stressed, I try not to pass it on. When I communicate to someone I am careful not to be short tempered or to say something hat would hurt someone's feelings.

It is also important to do something nurturing for yourself; take a yoga or movement class, have a bubble bath get a massage, take a walk or have a healing session such as Reiki. Most of all, don't be hard on yourself. If you feel depressed take the time to see what it is I your life that bothers you. Write down what you would like to change and what it would take to change it. Write the first step and how to make it happen.

How does yoga help you to look and feel young?

For me, yoga awakened the spiritual side of movement; it is the unity of mind, body, and spirit. I realized the importance of the breath and of moving one's energy through all your chakras. I experienced the joy of feeling the moments of unifying your spirit and body as a dynamic whole, as you connect to your eternal and sublime center.

What other activities do you enjoy?

I love learning new ways to move and have taken classes in ballet, modern, African,

Live Long, Look Young!

Haitian, Pilates, and Chi Gung. When I ski, I love the clear mountain air and gleaming white slopes. It inspires me to write a new symphony. Scuba diving and floating with the fish makes me marvel at nature's beauty and diversity. I also enjoy dancing with friends at a club.

All of these activities release stress and are wonderful social ways to exchange energy in healthful environments. In addition to stretching your muscles, activity also helps you to stretch your mind by pushing yourself to do new things. New challenges stimulate your brain. It keeps you in the here and now; you are inspired to create the next magic moment in your life.

Hair & Teeth

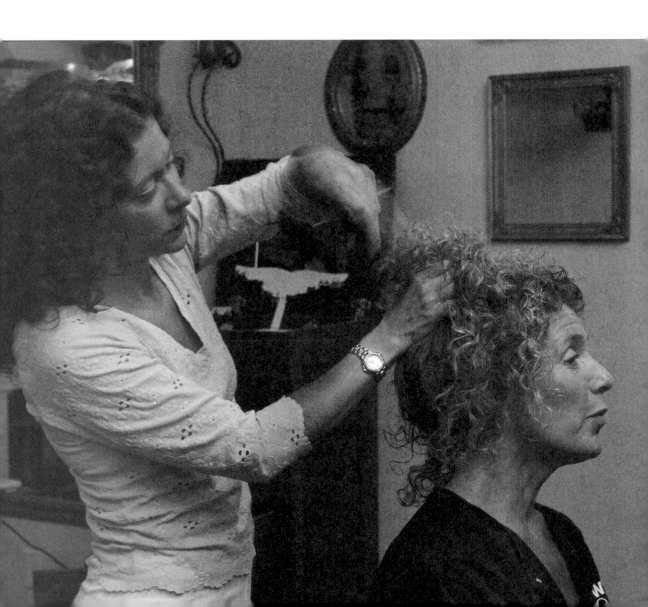

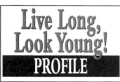

Live Long, Look Young! PROFILE Vicky Magliaro—41 years young—Licensed Beautician

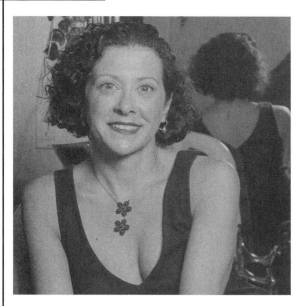

Vicky likes to tell it like it is. She is honest with the clients who come into her salon and expect miracles. "Please don't insist on something irrational; we are experts for a reason and we are looking out for you and will advise you on how to keep your hair in optimum health," she says. With 20 years of experience as a licensed beautician, she has seen it all. She acknowledges that while there are things that we simply cannot change, such as our genetics, there is a tremendous amount we can do in order to look and feel beautiful.

Hair care, of course is essential to Vicky and she recommends being gentle with your hair, frequently brushing and washing it. In her opinion, hair extensions are out as they do damage and color is a matter of preference. She recommends multi-shade coloring when hair is about sixty percent gray.

Vicky's expertise is not limited to hair care. She recommends facials for keeping skin free of pollutants as well as manicures and pedicures for those tell-tale age indicators: our hands and feet. And of course, a regular exercise routine is essential to combat the downward pull of gravity. Vicky has been active, participating in a variety of sports since she was a girl.

Above all, Vicky believes happiness will keep you young. "How many people are truly happy? Being happy is an essential part of living long and looking young. Forget that old wives tale—don't smile you will get lines. Be happy and smile."

Healthy Hair

In this section, Vicky Magliaro, a licensed beautician for over twenty years, provides some great advice for aging with grace and beauty; in particular how to keep your hair shiny and healthy:

Every day we wake up and face ourselves in the mirror and see what we all fear the most: growing older and facing difficult changes both inside and outside of our bodies. The good news is that there are many positive things we can do. The bad news is there are things we just cannot change. Luckily, esthetics can be altered to a large degree. Cosmetic surgery has been growing in leaps and bounds worldwide. We have many health spas and beauty salons that boast they can improve our appearance. Exercise gurus promise to trim the fat and make us mean, strong and lean. Yes, we are lucky.

Unfortunately, there are ugly truths that play a large role in the way we age that include genetics, illness, environmental hazards and unhealthy habits. We can undo some of the damage; it is never too late to take care of oneself. It is only too late for the dead and buried.

I always tell my parents, who live in Florida, that no one is holding a gun to their heads, forcing them to eat cake. Their idea of exercise is complaining that they need to lose weight. They claim they swim, but they don't even have bathing suits that fit! I can't understand how my parents managed to raise three extremely active, fit children. We were lucky and grew up in a neighborhood with plenty of kids and plenty of sports. I never remember a day without playing something. In the long run this has paid off. I have continued a lifetime of activity that has kept me in prime shape.

In the beauty industry we use scare tactics to sell our products and services. In actuality, we are trying to get you to maintain your looks. Everyone people watches and says "wow, doesn't she look great!" Well, everyone can look and feel great but it takes hard work. We all have our little secrets and tips, and are writing this book to share them with you.

Keeping our esthetics the best we can helps us feel so much better. As a licensed beautician for over twenty years with my own salon I suppose I qualify as an expert on the aging process: at least from the neck up! My first bit of advice is that you should put yourself in the hands of professionals. I have seen many undergo countless numbers of surgical procedures, which render their hairline way back behind their ears. Sometimes too much of a good thing does more harm than good. Eye lifts are great. They make you look younger and more awake. Eliminating the sags definitely takes off years—not to mention unwanted wrinkles.

Live Long, Look Young!

Let's move on to unwanted hair. As we age and our hormones change we end up with unwanted hair. Many women experience this after pregnancy when moles and hair seem to sprout everywhere. First, make sure you keep your eyebrows plucked and clean. Something as simple as a brow wax can take years off your looks (don't forget you can wax off those little hairs on your big toes too!). Chest hairs should be plucked. And, waxing any chin hairs will keep your face looking clean. Ladies, wax your facial hair. The more you wax the less it grows back.

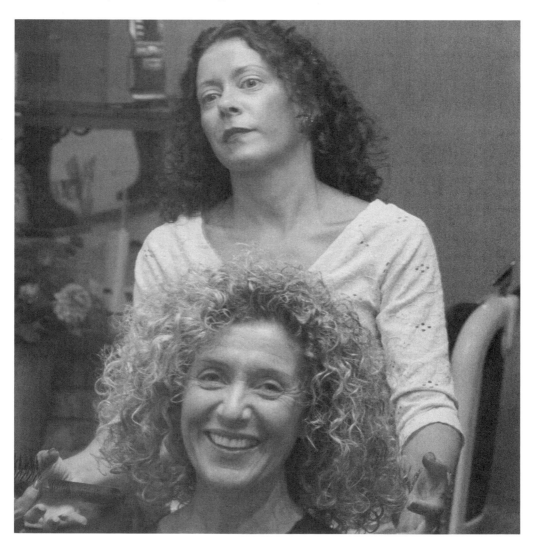

Care For Your Hair

We all want the same luxurious hair we had in high school. However, due to extreme hormonal changes in our bodies, that simply won't happen. We are lucky now that we are so advanced in the industry of hair color, styling products, chemical processes and skin care that we have an abundance of ammunition with which to combat the thinning and graying of our hair.

First, I have found that you must be ever so gentle with your hair. Treat it kindly with gentle pure shampoos and conditioners. When it comes to thinning, the good news is that many styles today are geared toward fine hair. Make sure you use conditioner for fine hair.

Brushing

Brushing is very important to maintain the shine and health of your hair. Use natural bristle brushes, which are gentler than plastic brushes. Soft paddle brushes with natural boar bristles are the best. Brush your hair before going to bed to distribute the natural oils, which help to naturally condition your hair. Remember the old days of brushing your hair 100 times before going to bed? It gave us the long, luxurious, shiny hair. Please brush.

Never rough up your hair with a towel after shampooing. This causes the cuticle layer to split. The cuticle layer resembles fish scales and when it is roughed up, it can be damaged. Wide-tooth combs are perfect for combing out your hair after shampooing. It is also a good idea to brush out your hair before you shampoo in order to distribute natural oils throughout your hair.

Shampooing

It is fine to shampoo your hair everyday. Use a gentle shampoo designed for frequent washing. Oily hair should be shampooed with a shampoo recommended for oily hair. There are remedies for every type of hair. Many men still believe that they shouldn't wash their hair everyday—that it will promote hair loss. But you can never be too clean and there is nothing nicer than clean hair. Make sure you condition as well. This is especially true if your hair is chemically treated.

Trimming and Styling

Trimming the ends of your hair every six to eight weeks keeps it healthy. You may also experiment with different styles. A change in style not only can make you feel better, but it can also take years off your looks. When we change our looks it gives us a whole new rush of excitement. A new haircut can lead you to change other things in your life as well: it may prompt you to buy a new outfit, new shoes, new make up, or even to find a new lover! There are so many fabulous looks that are forever resurging.

I know many women who are so lucky to have wonderful natural curly hair. What do they want to do to it? Straighten it. Why, I don't know. Chemical straightening is still popular but it does some serious damage to your hair, including breakage and loss of shine.

Women of color suffer the most from severe damage from chemical straightening because their hair is very fine and delicate. Fortunately, we do have much gentler products now for straightening. Using hot irons to straighten hair also causes damage. It is a good idea to use a product that protects hair from heat styling.

Another big trend these days, which is damaging hair is the use of hair extensions, which cause breakage, pulling, and thinning. They are a big money maker but trash your hair. I once had a client with naturally curly hair who proceeded to straighten it, highlight it, and weave extensions that were colored and permed into her own hair. This was a nightmare that was almost impossible to shampoo and comb out. Such stress can cause alopecia (balding). I strongly recommend against weaves. Make the best of what you have.

Coloring

Changing your hair color can make a great difference in looking younger. Warmer shades tend to soften our looks, whereas darker colors can be harsh. When selecting a color you need to keep in mind your skin tone and the amount of wrinkles that show. Dark colors will add shadow into cervices where light reflects. While it is generally recommended that women should lighten their hair as they get older, this is not always the best solution. Blond is not for everyone, especially since bleaching is so damaging to your hair. In addition, bleaching your hair blond over and over again lightens the hair so much that your roots will look darker than ever. Please don't insist on being a certain color if your hair stylist explains why it's not right for you. Remember that we are looking out for you and trying to keep your hair in optimum health.

You might want to consider highlighting your hair a shade or two lighter or darker than your own color. When hair starts to turn gray there are many shades throughout the head, which makes for a wonderful environment for highlighting. When hair is more than sixty percent gray it is the right time to try multi-shade coloring, which is more natural looking.

As far as gray hair in general, there are many women who are satisfied to keep their hair in its natural state. When gray hair becomes evident it takes on a whole new texture. Hair grays at different rates for everyone Loss of melanin starts the process and the hair lacks luster. Sometimes when hair starts to turn gray, it will become thicker. A semi-permanent color may restore the shine and condition. Where silver hair is shiny and soft, gray hair becomes coarse and wiry and needs more moisturizing products. Try using a clarifying shampoo and shimmer lights with a purple base in it to counteract any odd casts that gray hair can pick up. It will leave your color more brilliant.

Hair coloring for men is done much differently than for women. I usually use a deposit only low volume peroxide color for men because it keeps them looking natural. I also do think that men tend to look sophisticated with gray hair, whereas women tend to look older. If you are a balding man, I recommend letting it go gracefully and avoid combing over or wearing a toupee. Bald can be very sexy, hip and European (and it's way easier to maintain!)

Nutrition

Hair is the last source of protein in our bodies so if you deprive yourself of protein your body will rob it from your hair. Ridding your body of toxic waste will also keep all of you healthy, including your hair. Today we can perform a hair analysis to determine what toxins are present in our bodies. Anything that goes into your body goes into your hair. Drink plenty of purifying water.

Europeans have made wonderful contributions to the beauty industry. They are so much more advanced in hair care and skin care technology. They have wonderful product lines for thinning hair and natural products. Botanicals are probably the most popular.

Looking well groomed as we age becomes harder and harder but we have wonderful professionals to guide us through our golden years so that we can look the best that we can. I conclude my chapter with these few thoughts: Get out your lotions, creams, sun block, hats, antioxidants in every shape and form, jump ropes, roller blades, bicycles and dog (walking a dog is a great form of exercise.) Most important, be happy and enjoy life! Never give up your beauty because looking good is such a strong part of feeling good.

Your Smile

When you smile, you throw a little sunshine toward another person. As we age, we need to be extra diligent about caring for our teeth to ensure that we have the healthiest and best looking smile possible. Dr. Gerald Curatola, founder and director of East Hampton Dental Associates, P.C., a multidisciplinary dental group that focuses on integrative health and wellness, offers tips on how you can maximize your dental health:

Dental care today has come along way from the past belief that you should expect to "lose your teeth when you grow old." In fact, dentistry has taken the lead in promoting proper prevention and maintenance as the best ways to keep your teeth for a lifetime. During the past twenty five years, advances in technology have made it possible to not just make treatment more painless, but to also provide numerous aesthetic treatments for improving your smile—an important part of your physical appearance, self-image and spiritual wellness.

Prevention

- **USE GOOD ORAL HYGIENE:** As basic as this sounds, people on average spend less than a minute brushing their teeth, and most skip flossing—the only effective way to remove bacterial plaque between teeth. While all kinds of newfangled plaque-removing devices seem to arrive on the market each day, a good old-fashioned soft toothbrush and floss will still do the trick. But don't be cheap; it's recommended that you change your toothbrush every three to six months.

- **EAT HEALTHY:** Eating a diet rich in fruits and vegetables not only lowers your risk or oral cancer but provides vital antioxidants important for fighting all dental disease. Also, eat at regular periods. In between snacks, especially sugars and carbs, provide ammunition for bacteria and their acid by-products.

- **LIMIT ALCOHOL:** By having a dehydrating effect on oral tissues, alcohol strips both the teeth and gums of protective elements of saliva, promoting dental decay and periodontal gum) disease—the number one cause of tooth loss. Alcohol can also increase your risk of oral cancer.

- **AVOID TOBACCO:** In addition to the obvious cancer connection, all tobacco products accelerate advances in periodontal disease. Nicotine causes a strangulation of circulatory activity in oral tissues, promoting disease. In addition, tobacco causes a dulling of the sensory nerve endings on the tongue, causing diminished taste, as well as halitosis.

- **GET REGULAR DENTAL CHECKUPS:** The periodic dental examination on a three to six month basis not only screens for dental disease but can also diagnose signs of serious systemic diseases such as hypertension, diabetes, arteriosclerosis, AIDS, and cancer. The dental cleaning removes calculus and tartar below the gum line—this hardened mineralized plaque cannot be removed by a toothbrush.

Treatments

- **WHITENING:** With the use of carbamide peroxide or hydrogen peroxide, this simple procedure is both quite effective and affordable in turning back the clock with the color of your natural teeth. Teeth can be whitened by professionally administered at-home treatments or through an accelerated process in the dentist's office.

- **BONDING:** As a treatment for chipped, stained or worn teeth, the use of composite resin bonding materials placed and shaped directly onto the tooth's surface remains a low-expense aesthetic restorative choice. This procedure can also be completed in a single visit.

- **CROWNS:** With a wide range of new space-age ceramics, crowns are used to correct teeth weakened by decay, misalignment, and large old failing fillings. In addition, they are used to create a stable bite and improved aesthetics. Also fabricated in a dental laboratory, crowns are similar to veneers except that they cover the whole tooth.

- **INLAYS AND ONLAYS:** Fabricated from tooth-colored ceramic, composite resin, or gold, these restorations are used primarily to replace silver fillings. In addition to being very conservative to the natural tooth, they offer superior aesthetics and strength.

- **BRIDGES:** As a restorative treatment to replace missing teeth, bridges are placed on adjacent teeth to span the site of the missing tooth making this the treatment of choice to restore your bite as well as your smile.

- **IMPLANTS:** By using fixtures that are inserted into underlying bone to replace missing teeth, dental implants have given many patients, who previously were doomed to wearing dentures, another option. Once the implant is stable and integrated into the bone, a natural-looking crown is attached to the top of each implants, providing a predictable result of both function and aesthetics.

Natural Approaches to Dental Health

A number of nutritional, homeopathic and herbal remedies have proven to be effective in prevention, maintenance and treatment of various dental diseases. Among one of the most promising nutritional supplements is Coenzyme Q-10. While Co-Q-10 is highly effective topically on the gums, it also can be taken orally. Get the gel caps (rather than the capsules) for higher absorption, and take between ninety and one hundred twenty mg per day. Other supplements to take include Vitamins C, E, A and B-Complex, Folic Acid and Zinc. Homeopathic remedies include Arnica (for trauma, bruising), Calcarea Carbonica (strengthens bones), Calcarea Fluorica (a homeopathic form of fluoride, which strengthens teeth), Hepar Sulphuris (for gum infections), Hypericum (for dental nerve pain), Kali Muriaticum (for pyorrhea) and Pulsatilla (for toothache). While many other homeopathic remedies exist, a thorough diagnostic inventory is necessary before selecting one that is appropriate for you. Herbal therapies remain one of the oldest forms of medicine and have long been used in dental treatments. These include aloe vera, chamomile, cloves, goldenseal, myrrh, sage, tea tree oil, and wintergreen.

By following these preventive and treatment measures you can make sure your teeth and gums live long and look young for years to come.

six

Personal Development

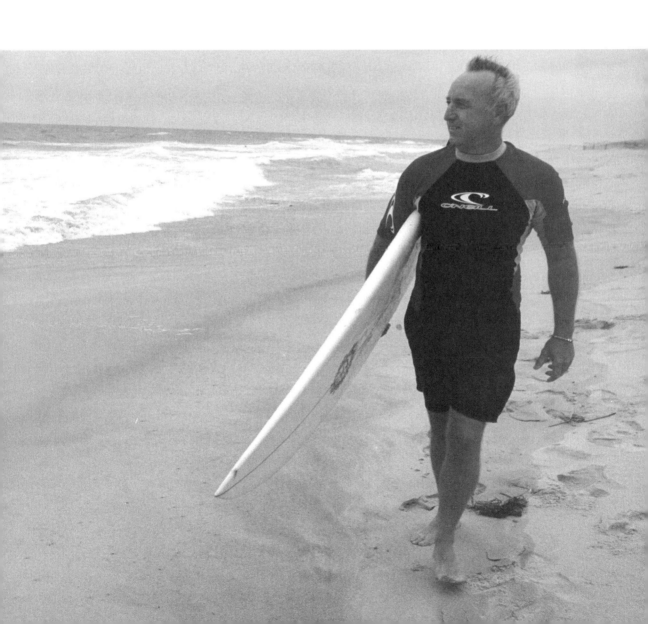

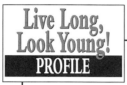 **PROFILE** | Jane Umanoff—58 years young—Prosperity Coach

"Tension and stress age people and are responsible for illness"

"I work with women and men who are interested in creating a balanced, fulfilling, joyful life," Jane says. 'They are interested in their personal well being and are open to eating and living healthfully, which entails exercise, yoga, and sometimes having a spiritual practice such as meditation." Jane recommends yoga to all of her clients to improve their general well being, relieve stress, attain proper alignment and breathing, and to experience the peace of mind and connectedness with the universe that a good yoga class elicits.

She also recommends that people continue to learn at all ages. "I believe I stay young and strong because I am open to new ideas," Jane explains. "I continually take classes of various sorts." She also eats a healthy diet, takes vitamins and herbs, exercises daily, stresses the positive in life and does yoga twice a week. It helps that she loves her work, her job and her family (which includes a new grandson).

"I relieve tension through yoga and meditating," Jane says. "I believe that tension and stress age people and are responsible for illness—or at least can influence the immune system."

Productivity

Sometimes it is difficult to feel that we are leading productive lives; being the best that we can so that we can set and accomplish new goals. We may be feeling out of balance, tired and dissatisfied with the way some things in our lives have turned out—whether they are our relationships or professional endeavors. Or, sometimes we simply want a positive change and need some direction. When this occurs, it may be helpful to contact a professional prosperity coach.

Jane Umanoff is a prosperity coach who works with individuals and couples on both personal and business matters. She uses coaching, which she calls goal and action oriented as well as therapy, which is feeling and healing oriented. "The foundation of my philosophy is around acceptance of self, to learn to tolerate ambivalent feelings, set standards, set boundaries, forgive ourselves and others, let go of judgment and to learn to act from our commitments rather than from or feelings," Jane explains.

Jane takes a holistic approach that includes both the mind and body, and uses psychodynamic as well as family systems theory; solution-focused psychotherapy, focusing, Feminist Relational Psychotherapy (a la Stone Center) and EMDR (eye movement desensitization and reprocessing). EMDR is a powerful new method of psychotherapy based on the observation that eye movements can reduce the intensity of disturbing thoughts under certain conditions. During EMDR the therapist works with the client to identify a specific problem to be worked on. Using bilateral stimulation through sets of eye movement or tapping, the client processes information and feelings Jane also uses meditation, some energy healing, and twelve-step work with her clients. She shares her multi-modal approach below:

"We begin by having a conversation about what the client wants to accomplish in therapy/coaching—what he or she envisions if our work together is successful. Next, we do a family map or genogram, which helps the client see family patterns, beliefs and themes. Then we begin to do the work of awareness and acceptance in the above-mentioned ways. It's important for all clients to know where they come from and then to begin to see that they have choices. It's very difficult to change unless we are aware of who we are and come to accept ourselves. A body/mind approach lets us get in touch with internal sensations, issues and feelings, and allows us to accept who we are. This is so important before we can change our behavior.

"Coaching is a helpful technique I use to foster new ways of behaving. The client has an opportunity to set new standards for behavior and then set boundaries. Our coach-

other aerobic exercise, psychotherapy, working with a coach, becoming a psychotherapist and a coach, being a mother and now a grandmother, forgiving my parents, my husband and my children, and listening and receiving from my good friends. The most forgiving thing I can do for myself and for others is to not judge—but to think and behave from my higher self— a way that lets me feel good.

"Forgiveness can also be a conscious change in attitude. When I am feeling resentful or angry towards another, I realize that usually hurts me more than anything else. And it is often held in the body unconsciously as chronic pain, fatigue, or isolation. To become aware of our feelings helps bring light to the situation. Once there is some breathing room for the feeling, there is the opportunity to shift from awareness to acceptance and forgiveness. I do this work for myself daily and work with my clients on it regularly. To illustrate this, two case examples follow:

"Frank and I have been working together for two years. Frank came to me for financial coaching, to get his finances in order and to decide his career path. He was not particularly interested in psychotherapy per se, but over the time we spent together, he slowly became aware of his feelings and body sensations and how they were a clue to his outward behavior. He allowed himself the time for some gentle exploration of these feelings and realized that his boundaries with his family and his employer were not self-supportive. We worked on boundary issues and he created a completely new relationship with his mother and siblings. He was earning a great deal of money and believed it was his responsibility to take care of his mother. Through our work together, he was able to lead a family meeting and empower his siblings to share the responsibility. This was a wonderful example of how Frank began to set standards for himself and then set boundaries. It also brought him into closer relationship with his siblings and mother. They became a more connected family. Frank is no longer the sole caretaker. Now he can focus on his own financial issues: getting paid appropriately for his incredible contribution at work, cleaning up old debts and beginning a savings program for his future. In the process, he began to take extremely good care of himself: morning walks, time for meditation or relaxxation, time for de-cluttering, and setting goals in alignment with his values—which for him meant writing and being published. Now we are working on his creating a career from his passion and desires and not from what he thought he *should* be doing.

"To manage the contact within relationships with people, places and things well is a way of taking care of ourselves, having integrity, and having a sense of freedom of action. I have spent much time, thought, and prayer or meditation in learning how to forgive myself. Awareness, acceptance, forgiveness, and action or change have been the main stepping stones on the path of my personal development, which has come about through so many means: my twelve-step program, yoga, meditation, walking and

ing relationship focuses on the client having a harmonious, balanced life in all its aspects: career, relationships, personal well-being, finance, environment and fun/adventure; it's not just about feeling happy, sad, anxious, angry, lonely, loving, etc. Coaching is a more active approach than therapy in creating a structure to support the actions the client wants to take. In the coaching process we stand in the future, looking back on this current year, creating a 'vision' of what we want. Out of the vision we set quarterly goals or intentions in each of the areas of life. I have clients make sure that these goals align with their values—so that they are coming from a place that's really important to them and not just checking off a to-do list."

Boundaries

"In taking extremely good care of ourselves, I think we must first look at incompletions in our life as well as what we are tolerating. When we create closure on open issues around finances, taking care of our home, and upsets in relationships we experience relief; what follows is an opening, and new energy to take on what we really want and value in our lives. Another way of creating personal well-being is to set standards that come from our higher self, from our quiet yet all-knowing intuition. The process of setting standards helps us distinguish between our own and other's acceptable and unacceptable actions, habits and behaviors. Once this is done we can set boundaries.

"A boundary is a line drawn all around us that prevents us from being influenced by others. Unlike walls, boundaries are flexible, changeable, removable, and semi-permeable. In his wonderful article *Know Your Boundaries*, Charles Whitfield explains that healthy boundaries are like healthy cells within our bodies. When the cell—a semi- permeable membrane—functions correctly, the cell wall keeps poisons out, let nutrients in, and excretes waste. It also defines the existence of the cell by separating it from other cells. Healthy cells show good contact at their boundaries by discriminating between nutrition and poison, and by positioning and duplicating themselves. The healthy client must learn to do the same. That means we have to learn when to allow people, ideas, etc. in and when to keep them out by setting healthy, roomy boundaries.

"To manage the contact within relationships with people, places and things well is a way of taking care of ourselves, having integrity, and having a sense of freedom of action. I have spent much time, thought, and prayer or meditation in learning how to forgive myself. Awareness, acceptance, forgiveness, and action or change have been the main stepping stones on the path of my personal development, which has come about through so many means: my 12-step program, yoga, meditation, walking and other aerobic exercise, psychotherapy, working with a coach, becoming a psychotherapist and a coach, being a mother and now a grandmother, forgiving my parents, my husband and my children, and listening and receiving from my good friends. The most forgiving thing I can do for myself and for others is to not judge—but to think and behave from my higher self—a way that lets me feel good.

"Forgiveness can also be a conscious change in attitude. When I am feeling resentful or angry towards another, I realize that usually hurts me more than anyone else. And it is often held in the body unconsciously as chronic pain, fatigue, or isolation. To become aware of our feelings helps bring light to the situation. Once there is some breathing room for the feeling, there is the opportunity to shift from awareness to acceptance and forgiveness. I do this work for myself daily and work with my clients on it regularly. To illustrate this, two case examples follow:

"Sally came into therapy feeling overworked and depressed. Focusing provided her with a way to become connected with her feelings and be gentle with them—not do anything but breathe and accept who she was in the moment. Focusing helped Sally release tight and uncomfortable feelings in her stomach and chest. She was able to explore her workaholic nature and what that was all about. Recently, she left her extremely stressful job to take a managing position in a more creative venture. She has already set boundaries with her employer by setting up her vacation schedule in advance. She has done some excellent work regarding her family setting excellent boundaries with her parents. She has done EMDR and that has given her a healthier perspective of her parents and her relationship with them. The genogram (family map) was also very helpful for Sally to see her life in the context of her nuclear and extended family. She could see where she comes from, what beliefs she would like to maintain, and what beliefs she wants to let go of. She has created a vision of family, work, and creating a warm, safe, comfy home in the Berkshires and a getaway in Provence. She is currently exploring relationships in her life. We continue to use focusing and will also include EMDR to heal past small traumas. People can continue to change and grow throughout their lives by looking inward."

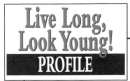

Frances Alenikoff—80 years young—
Dancer, Choreographer,, Artist and Writer

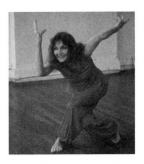

Frances is an inspiration to all who meet her. Many find it hard to believe she is eighty-years old. A dancer, choreographer, visual artist and writer, Frances has created more than ninety dance and theater works thus far in her career.

"I'm always looking for a new challenge," says Frances. "Some people zero in on one aesthetic and successfully make their name with it. I am always moving to the next thing, intrigued by new creative possibilities to explore. There are always more adventures, discoveries, and sensual delights on the way to keep our fires kindled, if we remain open and porous."

Frances believes that this attitude is what keeps her so young and vibrant.

When you drive up to her home you know instantly that you are in the presence of creativity. Outside there are rocks painted with all sorts of faces; on the walls of her dance studio are drawings of dancers and themes from the dances she has created in addition to many photographs of Frances performing. "One of the best gifts my passion for dance has given me is the enduring compulsion to stay attuned to the call and necessities of the body," she says.

In addition to all of her creative arts work, Frances has studied yoga and breath work, which she integrates into her dance. Frances feels that yoga enables you to be deeply in touch with yourself and the vital energy that nurtures creativity. She combines that exploratory sensing with dance and voice to create her dance theater pieces. "There are ways to storm the stereotypes of aging and to keep the body vital, vigorous and sensuous. It takes research, imagination, and attention. One can erode the tyranny of ageist belief systems that contaminate our vision of growing older by breaking the so-called rules: through self-invented, life-enhancing and self-empowering creative options."

"Consider this: care of the body is linked to care of the soul," she says. "Your spirit and creativity are unleashed when you take care of your body."

Friendship

We all need to have people in our lives with whom we can be close and share important conversations and feelings. Those people may be members of our families, our friends or acquaintances. With acquaintances we often share conversation and perhaps social activities. Then there are true friendships. We usually have fewer close friends than acquaintances.

A good friend is someone who always has a place in your heart—someone you can talk to anytime about anything that is on your mind. True friends understand each other, and are there for each other in good times and bad. A good friend will take the time out of his or her busy day to meet with you and talk with you, especially if you are going through a difficult time.

Think of something really healthy to do with your friends Take yoga or aquatics classes together. Or, meet at the gym for some aerobics or weight training. Working out with a friend adds to your motivation as well as makes the workout go faster!

Friendship is something to cherish in life. If a good friend moves away, make sure you stay in touch. Call and e-mail your friend. Plan to visit him or her. You can look at it as an excuse to travel. You have built up a friendship over time: an old friend knows your history, your feelings, your philosophy on life in a way that is precious and too dear to lose. Friendships revitalize your spirit. Stay in touch. Send holiday cards to all of your friends. Or, throw an annual party for all your friends.

I have a good friend whom I see mostly during the summer. She is a wonderful person and very social. Every week she hosts a beach party in which everyone who attends is asked to bring something—an hors d'oeuvre or bottle of wine. People who play musical instruments will often bring their instrument and play it during the party. Usually

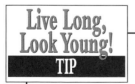

Being a Good Friend

Friends take turns listening to each other. Practice being an active listener.

the evening ends with the stars glistening overhead in the night sky, the bonfire roaring and people singing against the ocean's rhythm.

It is important to stay open to meeting new friends throughout your life. One way to find new friends is to engage in a social activity that you are interested in so that you can meet people with common interests. For example, occasionally I sign up for an art class. I love art and art history. Through these classes I always meet new and interesting people; sometimes friendships develop because we have common interests. Last year I went to Italy for the first time on a trip arranged by my art teacher. (To enable me to go, my husband and friends helped with the kids and I am very thankful to them). It was a fascinating trip! I truly loved Florence and, beyond the great experience of the trip itself, I met many new people with whom I shared good times. Today, I remain in contact with some of them, and we frequently share memories.

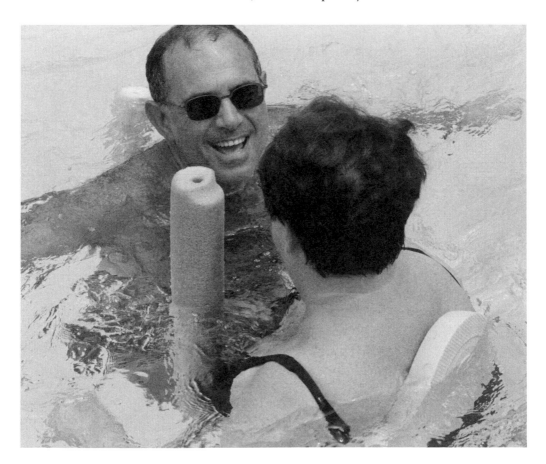

Live Long, Look Young! PROFILE Kent Klineman—68 years young—Lawyer, Venture Capitalist

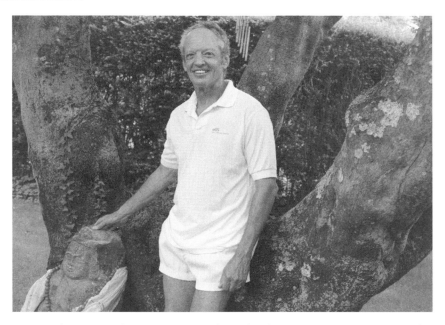

Kent is a lawyer and venture capitalist who loves action. His wife Hedy, an accomplished fine artist and he live in Manhattan and summer in the Hamptons on Long Island.

Seven years ago, Kent took up yoga, which he loves because he finds it calming. His secret to staying young and living life to its fullest is exercise and meditation. He gets a great deal of satisfaction from those practices and his work. He enjoys tennis, swimming, weight lifting and biking, and believes they keep him young. He also plays classical piano.

Kent is diabetic and uses exercise, meditation and love making with his wife to control his diabetes and live life with joy. He says it is also good to eat healthy foods and forget the booze.

"Staying in shape helps me stay balanced, alert and young," says Kent.

Love and Intimacy

It is important to nurture intimacy and care for close relationships throughout your life. These relationships can provide pleasure and security, and sustain you in times of need; they can encourage the setting and attainment of goals and the development of creativity. An intimate relationship must involve communication and support from both partners to allow the full growth possible for each individual.

If you find yourself with out an intimate partner, remember that it is never too late to develop a new relationship. However, before you look for, or give energy to a close relationship, look inside yourself and make sure that you are supporting and loving yourself. Throughout life, taking care of yourself is a continual process that will allow you to engender the resources needed to share love and energy with those close to you.

Sexuality is for adults of all ages to enjoy; that energetic attraction that pulls people together can be felt at any point in your life. When two people find themselves attracted to each other this is both exciting and healthy.

It is important for a couple to realize the benefits of taking time to relax together. You can do anything from taking long walks to sharing massage and practicing yoga together. These activities are very healthy; yoga increases circulation, reduces tension, and gets you in touch with your body and energy. Likewise, massage heightens your sense of touch and creates a wonderful feeling of sharing.

Sensuality and sexuality are important dimensions of intimacy. Sensuality can be expressed through touching, lying close together, massaging each other, bathing each other, and hugging. It can be a powerful and healing experience to simply lie close to your partner and breathe with them, gradually you may feel as if you are breathing as one.

Rekindle the sexual intimacy in your relationship by trying things such as new sexual positions, a romantic vacation, or aromatherapy. Try lighting candles, wearing a sexy outfit (this goes for both men and women), and watching a sexy movie. I suggest renting *Last Tango in Paris, Body Heat, or Bliss*. Everyone can increase the level of intimacy in their lives; it may be in the closeness of conversation or in the embrace of two lovers.

Breath…anchor to life
Movement…life itself
Sounds…embody the song of life.
Experiencing the fullness of our breath,
The sweetness of the inner dance,
The poignancy of the voice within…
We become porous to the depth and power
*   of knowing ourselves*
As a source and resource.

—Frances Alenikoff

seven

Emotional & Spiritual Development

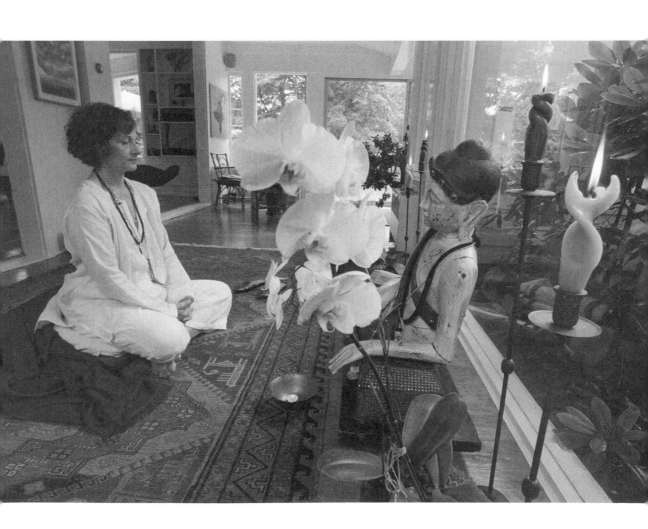

Attitude

Your attitude is very instrumental in keeping your mind and spirit young. Taking part in activities that you enjoy is very important. Take time to visit a museum or go to a show. Sign up for a course to learn a new language and plan a trip to that country.

Part of staying young is staying alert mentally, and not letting go of your curiosity about the world. Increase the time you spend doing the things that you love to do. Continue your hobbies or take up a new one.

I believe that if people really enjoy their work, they can continue working all their lives. (If a person doesn't want to retire) maybe they will want to change their hours, work at home or change their career all together.

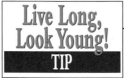

Strive to Feel Great...Often!

- Have as many positive thoughts and emotions as possible. If negativity comes into your life, realize it, deal with it, then try to let it go.

- Get to bed before midnight and wake up early.

- Get together with a friend you have not seen in a while. Maintain active correspondences through the phone, mail and e-mail with friends and relatives.

- Keep your living space light and cheerful.

- Give yourself body scrubs to rub off dead skin. Use natural creams, lotions and bath oils.

Live Long, Look Young!
PROFILE Jerry Starr—52 years young—Custom Builder/Surfer

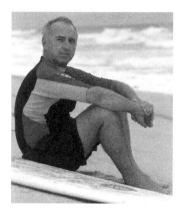

Jerry's secret to living well is moderation in everything that he does. "Excess in any form is what eats at your health," he says. "You can overdo anything whether it's food, drink, ambition, even exercise." Staying calm and eliminating excess stress also is all-important. The activities that give him the most enjoyment involve being in and around the ocean. Jerry loves to surf, bodysurf and swim, and this is perhaps the key to his youthfulness. Because he lives in the northeast, he can't be in the ocean all year long, so he travels to warm climates in the winter. Of course, traveling has its own rewards, which are adventure and coping with different situations and people.

Jerry has his own business with a partner. He is a very successful woodworker, building custom-made furniture for homes in the Hamptons and New York City. He considers his work a very important part of who he is, and he derives a great deal of satisfaction from it.

Exercise is one of the ways Jerry maintains good health and he strongly recommends it. "Try to do something physically stressful everyday. Take the stairs whenever you can or bike to the bank instead of driving," he advises. As for himself, Jerry surfs whenever there are waves. At the beach in the summer, he mixes in with surfers of all ages. The ocean is a medium in which they all feel comfortable. He also swims in a pool three or four times a week and stretches afterwards. Jerry recently bought a kayak, which he says is a great form of exercise. "I also spend time on resistance machines every week, which is very good for muscle tone," he adds.

Jerry feels that the fundamental theories of yoga are applied to all exercise. "In swimming when one is rhythmically moving, the yoga concepts of inhalation and exhalation, stretching and follow through are very much in evidence," he says. Jerry's outlook and health are an inspiration to surfers, woodworkers and to people of all ages.

Live Long, Look Young!

Our view of ourselves and our world are in a continuous process of change. We all pass through stages of birth, growth, maturity and old age. These stages are not rigidly defined. You can increase your health and youthfulness throughout your entire life!

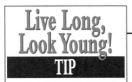

The Power of Positive Thinking

Norman Vincent Peale got it right. Think positively about yourself and you will be directed toward success. Believe in yourself and others will sense this confidence.

Think Positive

Positive thinking is a source of creativity and vision. In order to set and reach goals we need to believe in ourselves. There is very little room for pessimism—it zaps one of energy. Self-respect is the basis of positive thought. Give yourself a pat on the back whenever you can. Surround yourself with people who try to balance their lives, taking the whole person into consideration—body, mind and spirit. The highest level of thought is praise. Praise leads to peace, love and happiness, and encourages harmony and happiness. Positive thinking and relaxation go hand in hand.

Life works like a cycle. Positive thinking leads to positive action and feeling good about oneself. One thing that I really admire in people who remain ageless is the ability to change. Once your life becomes strictly routine, you rob yourself of surprise and creativity. If you are not afraid of change, your outlook on life will be more youthful.

Break Through the Restraints of Routine

Ask yourself how much of your life is spent mundanely because you are too lazy to try new things? Are you learning new things everyday? Does each day hold some significance to you? Do you have unfulfilled promises to yourself or others? Have you set a new goal and reached for it?

Wake up to new real needs. Fashion living patterns around these needs. Try more flexible patterns that leave room for creativity and spontaneity. Of course you need to have some routine in life. But try not to be ruled by routine. Question your living patterns for the week. This attitude will be reflected in your ability to avoid holding tension in your body, which of course improves circulation and posture. Yoga is very helpful in breaking down patterns of tension. Yoga teaches you to stretch and articulate all the muscles, tendons and ligaments in the body. A yoga workout moves circulation and energy through your entire body. Likewise, breaking hard-held patterns or routines helps to revitalize the circulation in your mind.

We can use positive visualization as a method of goal setting. By envisioning our ambitions, we make them more tangible.

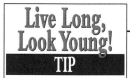

Try New Things

Keep the child inside of you alive. Be spontaneous—don't always go to the familiar.

Humor

Laughter is so important in life. Aren't we all attracted to people who can put a smile on our face? Unfortunately, so many of us take things too seriously. A part of being healthy is being able to let go of stress, making room for positive things to occur. Laughter releases stress and puts things into perspective. Sometimes, we find ourselves obsessing about a problem and laughter can help us to stop. A good joke brings you right into the moment. You cannot think about the past or worry about the future when you are laughing.

Live Long, Look Young!

Let's say you are in a very important meeting and feeling stressed and on overload. A little laughter can break the tension. Your thought process clears and you are free to think creatively. Tension blocks and inhibits circulation. When you laugh, tension is released—both mentally and physically. You have more creative positive energy and in turn you can make someone else smile. If you feel yourself getting a little angry about something, try putting a smile on your face and you will not stay angry for long because a smile on the outside has a positive effect on the way you feel on the inside.

People are attracted to someone who is happy and makes others smile. I'm not talking about going around with a false smile because this lacks truth; just try turning your mouth up and smile when you are feeling a little down and see how that truly makes you feel. It's usually contagious; when you smile, others around you feel better and they too smile. It's like sunshine.

Laughter also has beneficial physical effects. When we laugh our breath deepens and our muscles are gently shaken; giving an internal massage to the muscles of the abdomen. When you let yourself go and allow a deep belly laugh you are toning the muscles in your abdomen as well. As you laugh you release tension in your solar plexus and start to breathe more fully; you also release tension in your face. Did you ever see a person with a frozen expression? Someone needs to go over and tickle him or her!

There are so many ways you can bring humor into your life, especially if you are feeling a bit down or depressed. Go to a comedy club and take in a great, funny act. You'll forget your cares for a few hours. Check out the latest funny movie, or rent one (Make sure you select one from the comedy section, no tear-jerker dramas!) There are so many great, comical books that will have you laughing out loud while you read; why not pick one up? And never forget the power of talking to a good friend who can help you see the lighter side of life.

There are times when we need to take things seriously and there are times to take things lightly. Laughter helps us to lighten up. We want and need to feel a full range of emotions in our lives. Being able to do this helps us to stay and look young.

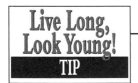

What's Funny To You?

Take note of what makes you smile and laugh. Movies, books, friends… and surround yourself with what makes you happy.

Guided Relaxation, Meditation and Visualization

Taking the time out to focus on relaxation will increase your sense of well-being and leave you in a calm, centered state. Yoga itself helps us to center ourselves; guided relaxation deepens this process. When you go into a deep relaxation after a yoga class you release blockages and allow your body to let go. As your body relaxes, so does your mind. Relaxation is a form of healing and rejuvenation.

During a guided relaxation, energy is balanced in your muscles, nerves and organs. Excess energy (Qi) is channeled from areas that are too full to areas that require energy. In this way, the body is healing itself. Try the following guided relaxation and enjoy the benefits of increased energy, and spiritual and emotional enrichment. You may find that when you first start doing guided relaxations that you actually fall asleep! This is common when someone begins because your body releases tension that it has been holding for so long. With experience, you will be able to stay conscious but be on the rim of the subconscious. Guided relaxation is not a passive act; it is a finely developed skill!

Guided Relaxation

You'll need to set aside ten to twenty minutes for this relaxation. Make sure you are in a quiet place where there are no disturbances.

Relax on your back with your eyes closed. If you have an eye pillow, place it over your eyes. Take long deep breaths into your lower abdominal area (also called hara) and release into gravity. Feel the weight of your body release. Travel through your body, releasing tension along the way. Feel your facial muscles let go, relax any fixed expression. Feel the relaxation as you release your jaw muscles and the tension in the back of your neck. Now let your upper back release into gravity and feel an opening across your chest. Tune into your breath as your rib cage relaxes. Feel your middle back release tension. Bring your awareness to your lower back. Feel the muscles on both sides of your spine release. Notice the circulation traveling through your hips and down your legs into your feet. Focus on your breath. As you inhale your stomach should rise and as you exhale it should lower.

You may feel that you can drift off to sleep. Stay in touch with the sensations you are feeling. This state can be called the yogic sleep. Just a few minutes in this space can rejuvenate you. As you travel through your body, notice if any areas still feel blocked or tight and use the breath visualization on page 5 to release tension.

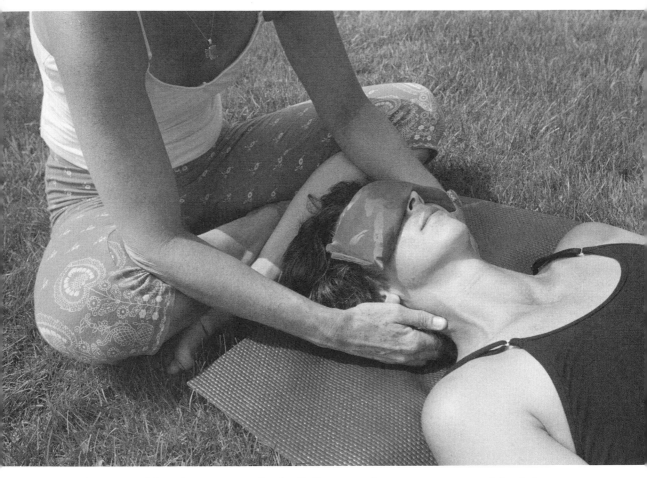

Come out of the relaxation very slowly. Roll to one side, open your eyes and slowly leverage up to a seated position.

You can practice relaxation techniques when you have time to rejuvenate. It is especially beneficial after exercise or before you go to sleep. It enables you to notice how good you are feeling from your activity; the benefits have time to sink in. Leave some time after your workouts, especially yoga, to experience the deep relaxation. The benefits of relaxation are just as important as the benefits of the yoga poses; there is a lot of rejuvenating and healing going on during the relaxation.

Meditation

Meditation can be done anywhere. I feel it is best to start meditating lying down as part of a guided relaxation or while sitting comfortably in a cross-legged position. The more you practice yoga the easier it will be to sit cross-legged. If it is difficult to sit up straight, place a pillow under your sit bones.

Meditation and relaxation go hand in hand. In most yoga classes the sequence is to go from the poses to a guided relaxation and then to end a class with meditation. It is very easy to enter into meditation after practicing yoga because you are already aware of the subtle sensations inside your body. Your mind and body are more relaxed and you can tune into your energy. As in yoga, when you meditate you are centered in the here and now, not thinking or planning.

So it is ideal to practice some yoga or go for a walk before you begin to meditate. If you are unfamiliar with the idea of meditation, another way of thinking of it is as contemplation. You abandon tensions in order to arrive at a creative, quiet place. Try to choose a place to meditate that is free from distractions. Begin by tuning into how you are feeling. Become conscious of your three-part breath. Throughout the meditation inhale through your nose; hold at the top of your breath, and then slowly exhale through your nose.

There are several benefits to meditation. It can help you do all of the following: develop an internal calmness, stability and clarity; tap into your creative side (after meditation you'll experience a surge in creativity); sharpen your intuition; achieve more fulfillment from life; feel refreshed; respond to stress with strength and flexibility; achieve a mind/body balance by looking inward. Many students find that guided relaxation and meditation are healing and help them to maintain good health.

One meditation that I often teach at the end of a yoga class or during a reflexology treatment is the Chakra meditation. During a Chakra meditation you visualize colors to help you focus your energy on various parts of your body. Chakras are energy points in your body that you create with your imagination, through yoga and visualization. There are seven Chakras in the body; the first is in the center of the pelvic floor, the second slightly under the belly, the third in the solar plexus region, the fourth in the center of your chest, the fifth in the middle of your throat, the sixth in-between your eyes and the seventh at the crown of your head. Each of these can correspond to a color in the rainbow: red, orange, yellow green, blue, indigo and violet.

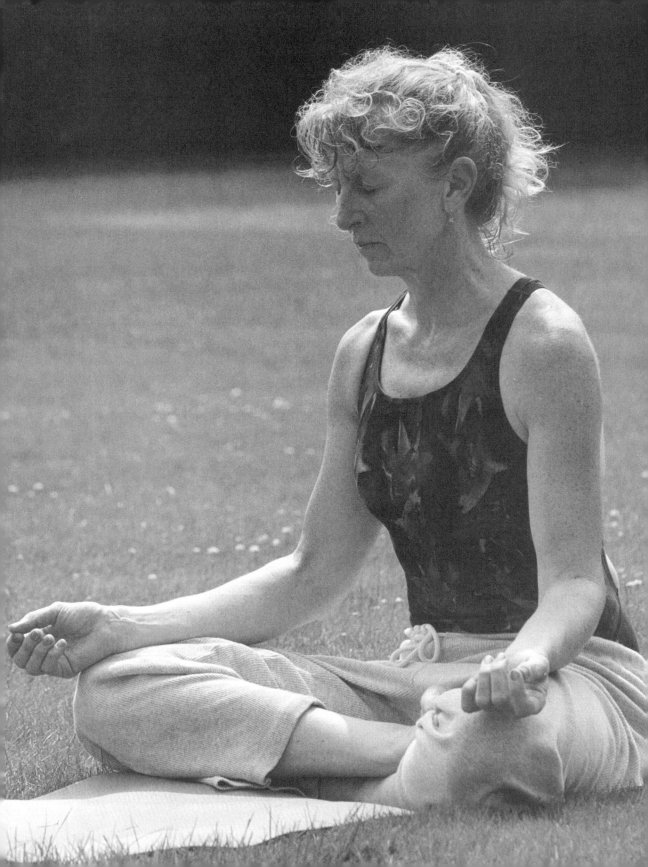

Here is an example of a Chakra meditation:

RED: Lying or sitting comfortably, feel the circulation move up the front of your body as you inhale and down the back of your body as you exhale. With each breath tension is being washed away. Tune into your pelvic floor and think of the color red traveling through your pelvis, moving toward your lower back and through your pelvic floor and around your hip sockets.

ORANGE: Imagine the color as a liquid traveling up towards your belly button turning into orange as it moves in between your belly button and lower back, then moving inside your torso around your waist sending healing energy to your back and stomach.

YELLOW: Focus on your solar plexus area, which is your body's energy center—your upper abdomen, behind your stomach. Imagine a shining golden yellow light radiating from the center of your solar plexus in all directions releasing tension from the center of your torso and encouraging full breathing. As you inhale, feel your stomach expand and as you exhale feel it coming back in.

GREEN: Now feel the energy move towards your lungs. Think of green as you inhale and a darker green as you exhale. Feel your lungs expand three-dimensionally from the bottom throughout the middle and to the top. Each healthy breath releases tension in between your ribs and through your upper back.

BLUE: As you travel up toward your neck, see the color blue appear, spiraling slowly up your neck to the top of the first thoracic vertebra and then spiraling down to the seventh cervical vertebra. As you travel through the meditation let the hues of blue change.

INDIGO: See the lavenders and purples travel through your head, face and scalp, releasing excess energy around your face and scalp.

WHITE: See a violet and white light at the top of your head and feel that white light shower you with relaxation ad rejuvenation.

A Chakra meditation is very beneficial because it gives you the tangible tools of color to work with. Many people, especially artists, find a color meditation very easy to imagine. Others may require some practice to feel comfortable using colors. It may help to think of the spectrum of the rainbow when you are starting out.

Live Long, Look Young! PROFILE | Hedy Klineman—62 years young—Artist

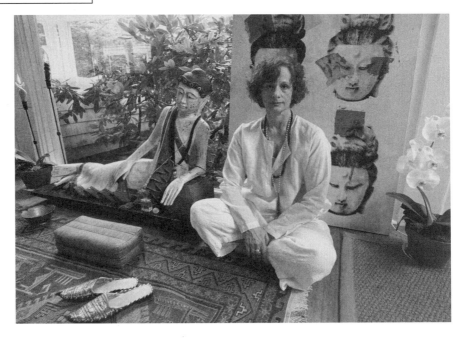

Hedy's secrets to staying young are meditation, chanting and yoga, and she funnels much of the energy from those practices into her art. "I am blessed to be able to work at what I love, the creative process is inspiring and fun," says Hedy.

Hedy began practicing yoga in the early 90's and she credits it with starting her on a spiritual path. She started collecting sculptures of the Far Eastern deities for her altar. Pretty soon, these images found their way into her paintings. For the past ten years, Hedy has been creating and showing this body of work, which she calls "Art and Spirit."

She goes to retreats at an ashram in Oregon several times a year to further deepen her connections to her higher self with yoga, meditation and chanting.

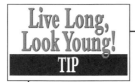

Chant Your Dreams True

Give yourself a dose of positive affirmation by focusing in on a goal that you have. Form it into a sentence and repeat it to yourself over and over. Then, file it away in your subconscious until you need to focus on it again.

Visualization

Visualization helps us to clarify our goals and file them into the subconscious. We do not want to become too attached to a goal because this leads to obsession and possible disappointment. In visualization, you picture a goal and if it does not happen right away, you try again at some point—perhaps taking a different approach. The thought that may come to you may develop into your next creative idea.

For example, I have been in the health field working on many creative projects over the years. I came up with the idea of a guided relaxation tape, which I produced. However, I didn't get the chance to market it so I put it on the back burner and didn't obsess over that idea. Then I met the publisher of this book and my series of yoga books, and was able to incorporate the idea of relaxation into this book. While my visualized goal may not have happened right away, the path I was on led to a related project. What next?

Creative visualization is a form of positive thinking. Envisioning your goal makes it more tangible and strengthens your motivation. Here's how to do a visualization:

Close your eyes while seated or lying comfortably. Feel your body float. Get to the place where you are just about to fall asleep but are still totally aware of what is going on inside you. Think of a goal that you are working on. Really picture yourself achieving that goal. For example, you may be trying to master a yoga pose. For me recently it has been the headstand. I knew I was ready to do it physically but something was holding me back. I practiced gently and regularly. I also visualized myself in the pose. I was patient and did not give up. One day, I was able to do a headstand and it really feels great! On to the next challenging pose…

Try to do this for yourself after a yoga class or yoga workout on your own. Do a guided relaxation and then visualize a picture of yourself in your mind's eye right across your forehead. Choose a pose that seems challenging. See yourself clearly doing the pose correctly and feeling all the benefits. Hold the image as long as you want to, seeing it clearly. Then, file it into your subconscious. The next time you practice yoga, try the pose again.

Other examples of creative visualization are emotional, creative, business or personal issues that you are working on in your life. Visualize one goal at a time. In a very relaxed state close your eyes and see yourself (and any other people in the visualization) clearly achieving your goal. Visualize it in color with as much detail as possible, then file it into your subconscious. Once you've filed it away it is stored for retrieval any time you want to see it again. You can always change or update a picture, or create a new one. A visualization is there for reinforcement and encouragement. Try to do a few relaxations a day if you are visualizing different things.

Another great example of using creative visualizations is in the sports world. Today, all athletes take time to visualize their event and a certain technique or play they have been working on. If a person is an Olympic athlete, he or she might see himself or herself pole-vaulting in perfect form at a desired height. If you are a golfer, you might envision yourself playing a certain way. Or, you may be a walker visualizing yourself walking along the beach on a bright sunny day, your muscles toned and your lungs and heart getting a healthy workout. You may see yourself becoming healthier and stronger.

In fact, visualization often is used to affirm health in what is known as a health affirmation. This is when you combine positive thought with visual images. Let's say you have a tightness or blockage in a certain area, such as a muscle spasm. Close your eyes and see this area as a place that is dark and needs more circulation. Go to that physical place with your imagination. Do a breath visualization described in the breathing section and see increased circulation in that area. Bring light and healing to that place.

We need to visualize ourselves as rightfully powerful and important—at any age. Our deepest fear is not that we are inadequate. Our deepest fear is that we are powerful beyond measure. It is our light, not our darkness that most frightens us. We ask ourselves, "Who am I to be brilliant, gorgeous, talented and fabulous?" Actually who are you not to be? You are a child of God. Your playing small doesn't serve the world. There's nothing enlightened about shrinking so that other people won't feel insecure around you. We are all meant to shine as children do. We are born to make manifest the glory of god that is within us. It's not just in some of us. It is in everyone and as we let our own light shine, we unconsciously give other people permission to do the same. As we are liberated from our own fear, our presence automatically liberates others.

Learn the techniques of guided relaxation, Chakra meditation and visualization and, like yoga, you will gain benefits that stay with you because you have integrated your body, mind and spirit.

Faith

Nourishing your spirit gives you the joy, peace and fulfillment that we all seek in life. Just as you make sure that you eat the right foods, get enough exercise and take care of your outer appearance, you need to tend to your inner self through meditation, and relaxation—as we've already discussed—and also by cultivating a spiritual life.

Susyn Reeve, an inter-faith minister in Sag Harbor, New York, has witnessed the great gifts that a spiritual foundation provides, and she credits her regular spiritual practice with keeping her young, for it provides her with a sense of "wholeness" which she says, "is an important component of my feeling a sense of vitality and radiance."

Tending to your spiritual life does not necessarily mean going to a traditional religious service, although it may. According to Susyn the important element is to create a spiritual practice, something that you do that nourishes your spirit and which enables you to feel whole and connected to something larger than yourself. For example, think about how you feel when looking at a beautiful fiery sunset, seeing a newborn baby, observing a full moon, or listening to a favorite musical composition. Often such moments fill us with a sense of awe and fullness and put us in touch with our spirit. How, then do you create your own spiritual practice?

Susyn recommends beginning with the *intention* to create a spiritual practice. You need to really want to evolve your spirit. Then, choose a place that is conducive for you to feel the presence of your spirit, and create an altar there. Perhaps this will be your favorite room in your house. Susyn has a altar in her living room upon which she places things that speak to her spirit: candles, photos of loved ones, a feather, a shell, a stone that she found a beach. "When I look at my altar I often sigh into a sense of calm and I often meditate facing it,"she explains.

Once you have created this spiritual place, commit yourself to experimenting for forty days with a specific practice. You may meditate daily, read and reflect upon an inspirational passage, write in your journal, converse with God, or ask a question and listen to the still, small voice within you. Susyn's regular practice includes reading an inspirational passage each morning and evening, meditating fifteen minutes each day, writing in her journal, praying, and before going to sleep making a list of all for which she is grateful.

These practices provide Susyn with guidance that helps her in difficult situations, whether they are serious problems like illness of loved ones or frustrating situations such as being stuck in traffic jams. In these situations, she says she is "more apt to hear the still small voice within calling to me" and she can respond in faith and love, which provides a vitality and radiance from the inside out.

177

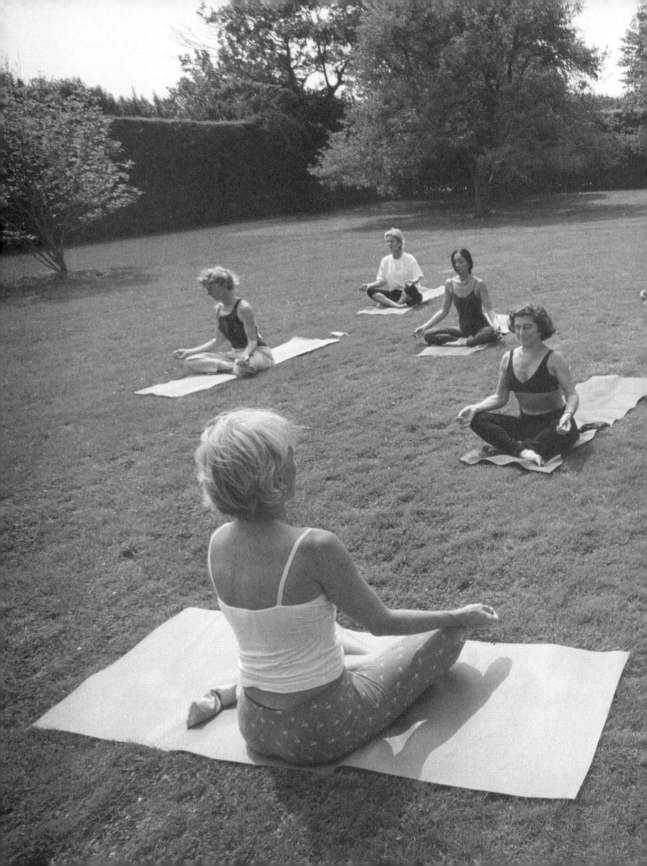

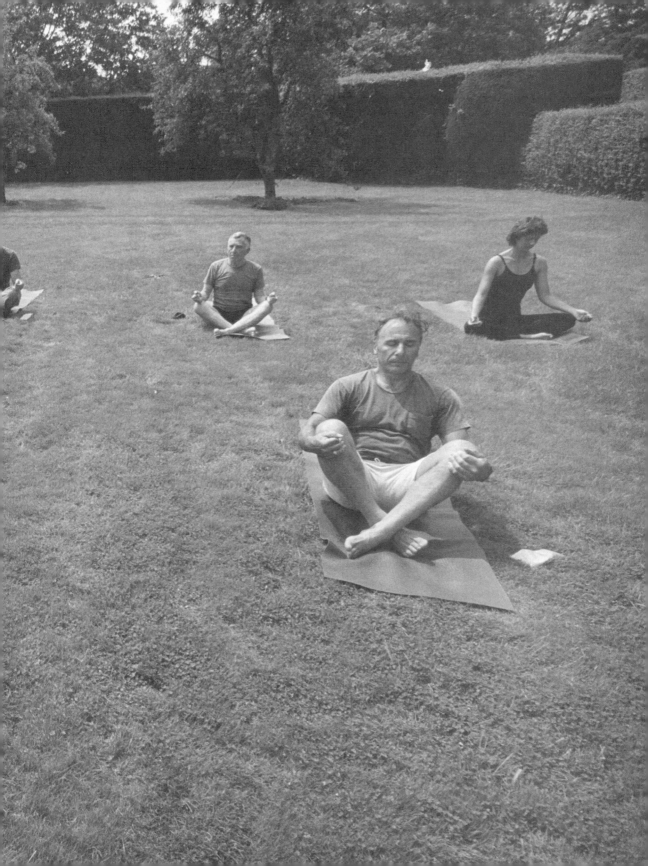

Live Long, Look Young! PROFILE

Susyn Reeve—52 years young*—Inter-Faith Minister

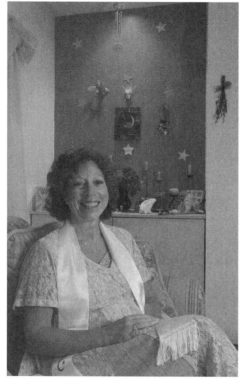

For the past twenty years Susyn has been a consultant focusing on organizational and personal development with clients that have included Mount Sinai, Montefiore Medical Center, Exxon, and Continental Airlines as well as individuals. She has helped her clients to clarify goals, reduce stress and communicate more effectively. Often, she found when working with her clients the importance of a spiritual perspective.

Today she is a candidate for ordination as an inter-faith minister and leads an inter-faith Sunday Service in Sag Harbor, New York, that focuses on creating and nourishing a community of faith, and supporting and guiding people on their journey of faith. She also does individual counseling with a spiritual perspective and leads a weekly Living Enrichment Circle to support people in practicing spiritual principles as the foundation of their daily lives.

A "Spiritual Seeker" for nearly thirty years, Susyn recommends yoga as a way to connect the body, mind and spirit. "Yoga is a powerful method to engage the body/mind/spirit," she says. "Too often in spiritual practice people have the tendency to exclude their bodies. A full experience of vitality must incorporate all aspects of our humanness."

To relieve tension, which she believes ages a person because it creates a focus and perspective that revolves around fear, Susyn recommends the following:

prayer, meditation, physical exercise, talking with a good friend, writing in a journal, focusing on what you are grateful for, doing yoga, being in nature and playing.

Susyn credits her regular spiritual practice, which consists of mediation, reflection, prayer and journaling, with her youthful appearance and vitality. "The inner glow from my regular spiritual practice gives me the energy to nurture my physical and emotional life. My connection with God, the energy of Love in the Universe, provides me with the knowledge that each situation and circumstance in my life carries a gift in it, even though it might not be apparent at the moment. My spiritual connection prompts me to ask the question "What would Love do here?" when faced with difficulties. When I listen to the answer and put it into practice, I see the world through a loving perspective rather than a fearful one.

One of Susyn's favorite spiritual practices is to take a bath. "Before I get into the tub I light two candles. As I light the fist one I say: 'This light symbolizes the presence of God—the energy of Love which is always present and available in and through me, in all that I am, have and do.' As I light the second candle I say 'This light represents the full manifestation of my dreams.' Simply focusing my thought in this way enables me to feel a greater sense of connection."

In the Mayan tradition, fifty-two is the age at which we become adult.

Live Long, Look Young!

In addition to these spiritual practices, I see yoga and massage as great nourishment for the spirit. And enlivening the spirit is what all faiths have in common. The origins of yoga date back thousands of years ago to India, and the practice of it is very much intertwined with Buddhism. When we practice yoga we integrate our body, mind and spirit. After yoga we feel more centered and calm, and we let go of our ego.

Every Sunday morning I teach yoga while some of my friends go to church and others choose to be in nature. All of these are ways in which you can get in touch with your spirit and the spirit of others.

From the Teaching of Buddha

Master your senses
what you taste and smell,
what you see, and what you hear

In all things be a master
of what you do and say and think
Be free

Are you quiet?
quieten your body
quieten your mind

By your efforts
awaken yourself, watch yourself
and live joyfully

Create a Spa Program at Home

Sample Live Long, Look Young Programs

The different ideas and techniques for living long and looking young presented in this book may sound great to you, but you may wonder how you can combine them all into a manageable plan. Here are a couple of sample plans that you can use as guidelines when creating your own healthy living program. The key is to find a plan that you can maintain and enjoy; one that will de-stress and revitalize your body, mind, and spirit!

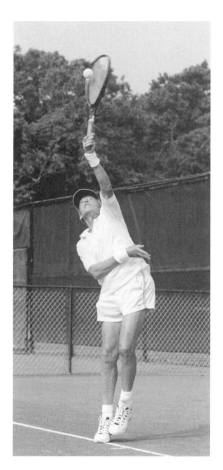

Plan A

	Sunday	Monday	Tuesday	Wednesday
Week One	Yoga Class: 1 hr. Walk: 20 min.	Walk: 20 min. Weight: Train: 15 min.	Bike: 20 min. Yoga: 10 min.	Walk: 20 min. Massage: 1 hour
Week Two	Bike: 30 min. Reflexology: 45 min.	Walk: 20 min. Yoga Class: 1 hour	Water Exercise: 45 min. Self-Massage: 10 min.	Seated Yoga 15 min. Walk: 4 min.

	Thursday	Friday	Saturday
Week One	Dynabands: 15 min. 10 min. Yoga: 15 min.	Facial: Exercise:. 10 min. Facial: 45 min.	Water: Exercise: 45 min. Tennis: 1 hour
Week Two	Yoga: 20 min. Guided Relaxation/ Visualization: 45 min.	Weight: Train: 20 min. Yoga: 10 min.	Yoga: 30 min. Dynabands: 15 min.

Plan B

	Sunday	Monday	Tuesday	Wednesday
Week One	Weight Train: 20 min. Walk: 30 min.	Walk: 20 min. Yoga: 1 hour	Bike: 20 min. Reflexology: 30 min.	Walk: 20 min. Dynabands: 20 min.
Week Two	Bike: 30 min. Yoga: 30 min	Walk: 20 min. Weight Train: 30 min.	Dance Class: 45 min Self Facial Exercise: 15 min.	Massage: 1 hour Yoga: 20 min.

	Thursday	Friday	Saturday
Week One	Water Exercise: 30 min. Yoga: 30 min.	Walk: 20 min. Self-Massage: 15 min.	Meditation: 20min. Yoga: 1 hour
Week Two	Walk: 20 min. Yoga Exercise: 20 min.	Weight Train: 20 min. Guided Relaxation/ Visualization: 20 min.	Yoga: 30 min Yoga: 20 min.

Resources

Aquatic Exercises

AQUATIC EXERCISE ASSOCIATION
P.O.Box 1609
Nokomis, Florida 34274

Aromatherapy

NATIONAL ASSOCIATION FOR
HOLISTIC AROMATHERAPY
888-ASK-NAHA
www.naha.org

MOOD BEAUTY
Mail Order
P.O. Box 166 Mill Neck Road, N.Y. 11765
e-mail: Mood@optonline.net

Dental Care

Stay, Flora Parsa D.D.S. *The Complete Book of Dental Remedies.* (1996). Avery
Publishing Group.

Exercise (general)

GETFITNOW.COM
www.getfitnow.com
1-800-906-1234

AMERICAN COUNCIL ON EXERCISE
www.acefitness.org
1-800- 825-3636

Intimacy

SexFlex (2000). Hatherleigh Press, N.Y.
Available at www.getfitnow.com
1-800-906-1234

Nutrition

THE AMERICAN DIETETIC ASSOCIATION
www.eatright.org
1-800-366-1655)

Osteoporosis

Daniels, Diane. Exercises for Osteoporosis. (2000).
Hatherleigh Press, N.Y.
Available at www.getfitnow.com
1-800-906-1234

Reflexology

HOME OF REFLEXOLOGY
www.reflexology.org

MODERN INSTITUTE OF REFLEXOLOGY
www.reflexologyinstitute.com

Reiki (music)

GODDESS TRILOGY AND MUSIC
MEDITATIONS INFUSED WITH REIKI
Available at all major music stores and Amazon.com
Website: www.goddessmusic.com

GODDESS AWAKENING- VOL. 1
Music to energize your soul
Stimulating sensual world beat rhythms
Inspire passion in your daily life
Finalist in Crossroads 2000 New Age Music Awards

GODDESS CELESTIAL REALMS - VOL. 2
For meditation, body work, relaxation
Sensual undulating pulses
Soothing ethereal vocals and melodic curves
Finalist in New Age Voice: Meditation/Healing Music

GODDESS MYSTICAL VISIONS - VOL. 3
Guided visualizations for
Physical and spiritual rejuvenation
Exotic imagery to relax, refresh, to dream
COVR 2000 Visionary Award: Best Spoken Word Album

Reiki (centers)

LOVING TOUCH CENTER INTERNATIONAL
SCHOOL OF TRADITIONAL REIKI USA
1-800-LT CENTER

THE CENTER OF LIVING LIGHT USA
1-631-728-4173

Yoga

Trivell, Lisa. *I Can't Believe It's Yoga.* (1999).
Hatherleigh Press NY.
Available at www.getfitnow.com
1-800-906-1234

YOGA RESEARCH AND EDUCATION CENTER
www.yrec.org

DIRECTORY OF YOGA
www.yogadirectory.com

YOGA JOURNAL
2054 University Avenue
Berkeley, CA 94704

PARTNER YOGA
Cain Carrol
Lori Kimati
Rodale Books 2000

DOUBLE YOGA
Ganga White
Penguin Books 2000

JIVAMUKI YOGA CENTER
404 Lafayette Street 3rd Floor
N.Y. 10003

AROMATHERAPY
Using Essential Oils for Health and Beauty
Danielle Ryman
Portland house/windward
1986

Bibliography

Carroll, Cain & Kimata, Lori. (2000). *Partner Yoga*. Rodale Publishing.

Feurstein, George. (1996). *Yoga*. Shambala Publishing.

Gach, Reed, Michael & Marco, Carolyn. (1981). *Acu Yoga*. Japan Publishing.

George, Mike. (1998). *Learn to Relax*. Chronicle Books.

Lindle, M. June (ed.) (1995). *Aquatic Exercise Professional Manual*. The Aquatic Exercise Association.

Maggio, Carole. (1995). *Facercise*. The Berkley Publishing Group.

Ryman, Danielle. (1986). *Using Essential Oils for Health and Beauty*. Portland House Publishing.

Tiwari, Maya & Esko, Wendy. (1991). *Diet for Natural Beauty*. Japan Publications.

COQUILLE PUBLIC LIBRARY